THE COMPLETE GUIDE TO ATKINS DIET

AN EASY-TO-MAKE, LOW CARB DIET COOKBOOK AND MEAL PLAN FOR SUSTAINABLE WEIGHT LOSS, ENHANCE HDL CHOLESTEROL AND BOOST BRAIN HEALTH

CATHERINE JONES

Copyright Page

© 2023 Catherine Jones

Table of Contents

Chapter 1: UNDERSTANDING THE ATKINS APPROACH

Dr. Robert Atkins's low-carb eating plan, known as the Atkins Approach, focuses on changing the body's metabolism to induce weight loss. This approach focuses on limiting the amount of carbs consumed, especially during the early stages, in order to induce ketosis. Weight loss results from the body burning fat that has been accumulated as energy throughout this metabolic state. The method consists of four separate phases that are followed in order to stabilize a better eating pattern and gradually alter the diet in order to reach weight goals.

The harshest phase of the Atkins Approach, known as the Induction phase, requires participants to consume no more than 20–25 grams of carbohydrates each day. This drastic cut is intended to put the body into a fast-acting state of ketosis, in which fat, rather than carbs, becomes the body's main energy source. After that, the Balancing phase introduces a wider range of foods, such as nuts, low-carb vegetables, and modest amounts of some fruits, to help relax the limitations on carbohydrates. This stage continues until the person gets closer to their goal of losing weight.

Fine-tuning, the next phase, is more complex since it requires gradually increasing the amount of carbohydrates consumed in order to determine the upper limit that permits weight maintenance without causing weight growth. This stage depends on monitoring the body's reaction to gradually reintroducing carbohydrates. Lastly, the Maintenance phase seeks to maintain the weight loss over time by implementing a long-term, balanced, low-carb eating regimen.

Although many followers of the Atkins Approach have reported success with weight loss and better blood sugar control, the approach is not without its detractors. Critics express apprehensions regarding possible dietary deficits and the elevated consumption of saturated fats that are frequently linked to this methodology. It is advisable to speak with a healthcare provider before starting such a diet to be sure it is suitable for your particular needs and health concerns.

Introduction to Low-Carb Eating

Low-carb eating is a way of eating that emphasizes healthy fats, protein, and non-starchy veggies over large amounts of carbohydrates. Due to its potential for weight loss and health benefits—particularly in controlling blood sugar levels and certain medical conditions—this eating pattern has grown in popularity.

Reducing the intake of foods high in carbs, such as grains, sweets, starchy vegetables, and many processed meals, is the fundamental component of low-carb diet. When this happens, the body starts using fat that has been stored as fuel instead of relying as much on carbohydrates for energy. This change in metabolism frequently results in weight loss and can help prevent blood sugar rises.

Different low-carb diets are more or less rigorous. Certain diets, such as the ketogenic diet, drastically limit carbs in order to cause the body to enter a state of ketosis, when it burns fat for energy. Others emphasize complete, unprocessed foods and permit a moderate consumption of carbs from sources such as nuts, seeds, and some fruits.

Proponents of low-carbohydrate diets point out that it can enhance metabolic health markers including HDL ("good") cholesterol and triglyceride levels. Furthermore, some research indicates that it might aid in the management of diseases including metabolic syndrome and type 2 diabetes.

Critics of low-carb diets, however, point out that because some food groups are restricted, there may be dietary deficits, especially in fiber, vitamins, and minerals. For certain people, sustainability and long-term adherence can also be difficult.

Before beginning a low-carb eating plan, like with any dietary strategy, it is advised to speak with a healthcare provider, particularly for those who have underlying medical concerns. Making a low-carb diet that is balanced and tailored to each person's needs and tastes is essential to maximizing benefits and guaranteeing enough nutrition.

Benefits of the Atkins Diet

The low-carb Atkins Diet has gained popularity due to a number of possible advantages:

Weight Loss: A lot of people, especially during the early stages of the Atkins Diet, report experiencing noticeable weight loss. Restricting carbs causes the body to switch to burning fat stores for energy, which helps some people lose weight quickly.

Improved Blood Sugar Control: Cutting back on carbohydrates can help people with type 2 diabetes or insulin resistance maintain better blood sugar regulation. According to some research, low-carb diets like the Atkins one may improve insulin management.

Appetite Control: The Atkins Diet's high-protein and fat-rich foods may help with appetite control by promoting feelings of fullness and lowering hunger, which may lead to a decrease in total food intake.

Triglyceride Reduction: Atkins and other low-carb diets have been associated with lower blood levels of triglycerides, a form of fat. A lower risk of heart disease is linked to lowering triglycerides.

Improved HDL Cholesterol: According to some study, low-carb diets modeled after the Atkins diet can boost HDL ("good") cholesterol levels, which may be beneficial for heart health.

Better Blood Pressure: Adhering to an Atkins-style low-carb diet may result in improvements in blood pressure, which may lower the risk of heart disease and stroke.

Even though these possible advantages are frequently mentioned, individual outcomes may differ. The long-term viability of the Atkins Diet, possible nutrient deficits brought on by limiting food types, and discussions over the health effects of consuming a lot of saturated fat are some of the critiques leveled against the diet. It is advisable to seek medical advice prior to beginning any diet, including the Atkins diet, to verify that it is in line with personal health needs and objectives.

Science Behind Carb Restriction

Dietary carbohydrate restriction has been well researched, illuminating a number of scientific facets of this strategy:

Metabolic Shift to Ketosis: When the body is deprived of carbohydrates, it starts utilizing fat reserves instead of glucose as its main energy source. The liver changes fat into ketones, which the body and brain can use as an alternate energy source. This process is called ketosis.

Mechanisms of Weight Loss: Restricting carbohydrates frequently results in lower levels of insulin, the hormone that stores fat. Reduced insulin levels can help with weight loss and fat burning. Furthermore, low-carb diets frequently encourage feeling full, which may result in consuming less calories and consequent weight reduction.

Effect on Blood Sugar Levels: Blood sugar levels are immediately impacted by carbohydrates. Limiting carbohydrates can help blood sugar levels remain more steady, which is especially advantageous for those who have diabetes or insulin resistance. This strategy might enhance glycemic management and assist control insulin levels.

Lipid Profile Changes: Research indicates that low-carb diets can improve the lipid profile by raising levels of HDL ("good") cholesterol and lowering triglycerides. There is a lower chance of cardiovascular disease linked to these modifications.

Appetite Regulation: Diets low in carbohydrates, especially those heavy in protein and good fats, may affect hormones linked to hunger and fullness, improving control over appetite and possibly resulting in less food consumption.

Health illnesses: Studies suggest that limiting carbohydrates may be beneficial for a number of illnesses, such as metabolic syndrome, polycystic ovarian syndrome (PCOS), and epilepsy.

Although research indicates that cutting back on carbohydrates may have advantages, people react differently. Critics point out issues with the quality of fats ingested, possible vitamin inadequacies, and the long-term viability of extremely low-carb diets. Furthermore, research on the ideal carbohydrate restriction level for health and weight control is still ongoing. It is essential to seek advice from a healthcare practitioner prior to making large changes to one's carbohydrate intake, particularly for those who already have health concerns.

Chapter 2: STARTING YOUR ATKINS JOURNEY

To guarantee a smooth transition to this low-carb strategy, there are a few essential things to take while beginning your Atkins journey. Start by being familiar with the stages of the Atkins Diet, particularly the rigorous restriction of carbohydrates known as Induction, which is the first phase that leads to ketosis. Prior to starting, it's important to set specific goals for your health and weight. This will help customize the Atkins method to fit your unique requirements.

Planning meals becomes crucial; avoid high-carb items and concentrate on including protein sources, healthy fats, and low-carb veggies. To stay on track, stock your cupboard with Atkins-friendly products and schedule your meals in advance. Throughout the day, make it a priority to drink enough water to stay adequately hydrated.

It is best to speak with a medical professional or a certified dietitian before beginning, particularly if you have any underlying health issues. This consultation can guarantee that the diet is in line with your medical needs.

Last but not least, keeping an optimistic outlook and looking for help from internet forums or support groups can offer direction and inspiration along your Atkins journey. You may stay on track and get your intended health results by keeping an eye on your progress and making the required modifications.

Preparing for the Atkins Diet

To guarantee a seamless transition and position yourself for success, there are multiple steps involved in getting ready for the Atkins Diet:

Research and Education: Learn as much as you can about the Atkins Diet before you begin. Recognize its tenets, stages, and the kinds of meals that are permitted and prohibited at each stage. With this knowledge, you will be able to plan ahead and make wise decisions.

Health Assessment: If you are currently taking medication or have pre-existing medical conditions, you should think about speaking with a healthcare provider. It can be ensured that the diet is in line with your health needs and goals by talking through your plans with a physician or a qualified dietitian.

Organizing the Pantry: Get rid of processed and high-carb goods from your pantry and refrigerator. Load up on items that are recommended by Atkins, like fish, lean meats, low-carb veggies, nuts, seeds, and healthy oils. If permitted during your chosen phase, stock up on full-fat dairy as well.

Meal Planning: Make a weekly meal plan in advance. Look for meals that are Atkins-friendly, then make a shopping list based on what is permitted during your phase and the recipes you find. Making a food plan will help you stay on the diet and ward off temptations.

Hydration: Increase your water consumption to start concentrating on being well hydrated. In addition to being essential for good health generally, water can help control appetite and cravings, particularly in the early stages of a diet.

Support and Mindset: Get yourself mentally ready for the dietary adjustments. Recognize that there may be a time of transition while your body adjusts to a new dietary regimen. Seeking assistance from loved ones, friends, or Atkins Diet online forums can be a source of motivation and direction.

Monitoring Your Progress: Keeping a journal can help you keep track of your food intake, energy levels, weight fluctuations, and other health and well-being-related observations. You can make the required adjustments by using this tracking to better understand how your body reacts to the diet.

Supplements: You may think about taking supplements to fill in any possible nutrient shortfalls, depending on your dietary intake and phase. Speaking with a medical expert about this can help you select the right supplements.

You'll be more prepared to begin this dietary adventure, maybe realize its benefits, and minimize difficulties during the transition if you read up on the fundamentals of the Atkins Diet and prepare well.

Transitioning to Low-Carb Eating

A smooth transformation in dietary habits can be facilitated by taking some crucial steps when transitioning to a low-carb eating regimen. Start by familiarizing yourself with the fundamentals and recommendations of low-carb diet, including which foods are recommended and which should be limited or avoided.

Evaluate what you eat now and begin cutting back on high-carb items while consuming more protein, healthy fats, and non-starchy vegetables. Get rid of processed and high-carb goods from your pantry and refrigerator and replace them with low-carb options like lean meats, fish, nuts, seeds, and healthy oils.

In this change, meal planning is essential. Create meal plans that follow the low-carb philosophy and look into dishes that use these foods. Making a shopping list according to your meal plan makes it easier to adhere to your new dietary regimen by ensuring you have the necessary ingredients on hand.

During this shift, staying hydrated is crucial, so concentrate on drinking more water. As your body adjusts to the dietary changes, staying hydrated can help manage cravings and hunger in addition to supporting general health.

If you have unique dietary requirements or health issues, you should think about consulting a qualified dietitian or other healthcare provider for help. They can guarantee a safe transition to a low-carb eating pattern and provide advice specific to your condition.

Finally, keep an optimistic outlook during this change. Recognize that your body may need some time to adjust to the changes. During this transitional period, seeking support from friends, family, or online communities who follow a similar nutritional route can offer motivation and insightful advice. You can successfully make this transition to a low-carb lifestyle by monitoring your progress and adjusting as necessary.

Setting Goals and Expectations

Whether starting a low-carb regimen like the Atkins diet or a ketogenic diet, setting objectives and controlling expectations is essential. This is an explanation:

Realistic Goal Setting: Prior to beginning, establish specific, attainable objectives. Setting clear, quantifiable, and achievable goals is crucial for any health improvement, including weight loss, improved blood sugar regulation, enhanced energy, and general health improvement.

Both short-term and long-term objectives should be taken into account. While long-term goals can center on general health gains maintained over several months or years, short-term targets might include decreasing a certain amount of weight in a matter of weeks.

Realizing the Process: Acknowledge that it will take some time to get used to a new eating schedule. Have patience with yourself until your body gets used to the new routine. For example, weight loss may not occur as quickly as anticipated, particularly after the first phase.

Health Over Numbers: Although losing weight is a typical objective, give priority to general health enhancements. Pay attention to non-scale factors like increased mental clarity, better sleep, and more energy.

Flexibility & Adaptability: Have the willingness to modify your objectives and standards as you proceed. Not every technique will work for everyone, so if something isn't going as planned, be open to changing your plan or consulting a healthcare provider.

Non-Scale Victories: Celebrate and give credit for non-scale successes. These could include higher energy and concentration levels, lower cravings for harmful foods, and better blood sugar levels.

Lifestyle Adjustments: Recognize that sticking to a low-carb diet, or any diet plan, requires making long-term lifestyle adjustments. It's a long-term commitment to better eating habits rather than just a quick fix.

Monitoring Your Progress: Continually evaluate and chart your advancement toward your objectives. This could include measuring, tracking your weight, keeping a food diary, or recording improvements in other health indicators.

Setting sensible, all-encompassing goals and controlling expectations will increase your chances of maintaining motivation, making significant progress, and seeing long-term benefits from your low-carb journey.

Chapter 3: LOW-CARB NUTRITION

The Atkins Diet is a well-known low-carb eating strategy that places an emphasis on cutting back on carbohydrates while boosting healthy fats, proteins, and non-starchy veggies. Its approach is based on a phased strategy that starts with a strict Induction phase that drastically reduces carbohydrates in order to put the body into a state of ketosis. Carbs are progressively added back in later phases so that the body can adjust to different carbohydrate amounts.

The main components of the Atkins Diet include healthy fats from avocados, nuts, seeds, and oils, along with proteins from foods like meats, fish, and eggs. This emphasis on nutrition seeks to increase satiety, offer long-lasting energy, and lessen dependency on carbs as fuel. The main feature of the diet is its correlation with reduced weight, increased energy, and stable blood sugar levels by means of ketosis, a state in which the body starts burning fat that has been stored.

Critics scrutinize the Atkins Diet despite its lauded advantages. Potential nutritional shortages and discussions about maintaining large intakes of saturated fat, especially in some diet variations, are causes for concern. The Atkins Diet does, however, provide some flexibility, enabling people to adjust their carbohydrate intake to suit their responses and health goals. Strict ketogenic phases or more moderate carbohydrate decrease are also options.

It is essential to consult healthcare professionals before beginning the Atkins Diet due to its impact on eating habits and potential health implications. This is especially true for individuals who already have health concerns. While aiming for desired results, regular monitoring and modifications can guarantee that the diet is in line with each person's health demands.

Principles of the Atkins Diet

The Atkins Diet is based on a number of fundamental ideas that minimize carbohydrate intake to promote weight loss and enhance general health:

Carbohydrate Restriction: In order to induce a metabolic condition known as ketosis, the Atkins Diet places a high priority on limiting carbohydrate consumption, particularly during the early phases. This change in metabolism pushes the body to burn fat reserves rather than carbs as its primary energy source.

Phased Approach: It is organized in stages, with the stringent Induction phase (usually involving 20–25 grams of carbohydrates per day) as the first. Phases that follow progressively reintroduce carbohydrates, enabling participants to determine their carb tolerance while preserving weight loss.

Protein and Good Fats: The diet places a strong emphasis on eating foods high in protein, such as seafood, meat, and eggs, as well as foods high in healthy fats, such as avocados, nuts, seeds, and oils.

These nutrients are essential for supplying energy and encouraging fullness.

Weight Loss and Metabolic Effects: The Atkins Diet attempts to normalize blood sugar levels and promote weight loss by limiting carbohydrates. The body burns fat that has been accumulated when ketosis is induced, which may result in quick weight loss and increased energy.

Change Your Lifestyle Permanently: Rather than being seen as a temporary diet, the Atkins Diet encourages people to embrace a low-carb, sustainable lifestyle. It seeks to establish long-lasting eating pattern modifications to promote general health and weight control.

Flexibility and Customization: The diet's flexibility enables people to tailor their strategies in accordance with their unique circumstances and health objectives. This flexibility can be used to accommodate a variety of demands and tastes, from rigorous adherence to ketogenic phases to more moderate reductions in carbs.

These ideas serve as the cornerstone of the Atkins Diet, which encourages people to consume fewer carbohydrates, rely more on fats and proteins for energy, and perhaps lose weight and improve their health by following a flexible and progressive eating plan.

Choosing Atkins-Friendly Foods

Choosing foods that fit the low-carb diet's guiding principles and place an emphasis on proteins, healthy fats, and non-starchy veggies is known as an Atkins-friendly food selection.

Choose foods high in protein, such as fish, chicken, cattle, pig, eggs, and tofu. These are important meal components that supply vital nutrients and encourage fullness.

Add Good Fats: Use nuts (almonds, walnuts), seeds (chia, flaxseeds), avocados, olive oil, coconut oil, and fatty fish (salmon, mackerel) as well as other sources of healthy fats. These fats are necessary for the absorption of nutrients and energy.

Non-Starchy Vegetables: Give special attention to non-starchy veggies such as peppers, asparagus, broccoli, cauliflower, zucchini, and leafy greens (spinach, kale, and lettuce). These veggies are rich in fiber, vitamins, and minerals and low in carbohydrates.

Low-Carb Fruits: Choose low-carb fruits, like berries (strawberries, blueberries, raspberries), which are lower in sugar and higher in antioxidants than other fruits.

Full-Fat Dairy (in Moderation): A few Atkins diet variations permit full-fat dairy products, such as cheese, butter, and cream, in moderation. They supply vital fatty acids and calcium.

Eat Less heavy-Carb Foods: Steer clear of foods heavy in carbohydrates, such as processed foods, cereals, sweets, and starchy vegetables (like maize and potatoes). These don't follow the Atkins Diet's low-carb guidelines.

Examine the labels: Verify product labels to make sure they comply with the Atkins Diet's carbohydrate requirements. Be mindful of added sweets and processed foods that could impede your development.

Plan and Prepare: To make sure you have the correct components for meals and snacks, make shopping lists based on Atkins-approved foods. Meal planning ahead of time can support diet adherence.

Focusing on these Atkins-friendly food groups and paying attention to carb content will help people make decisions that uphold the Atkins Diet's tenets and encourage weight loss and improved health.

Crafting a Balanced Meal Plan

Using the Atkins Diet framework, creating a balanced meal plan entails carefully choosing low-carb meals that nonetheless provide vital nutrients:

Protein Sources: Give first priority to foods high in protein, such as eggs, tofu, fatty fish (salmon, mackerel), lean meats (turkey, chicken), and plant-based proteins. These foods form the basis of meals because they provide essential amino acids and support the health of muscles.

Healthy Fats: Consume fats that are good for you, such as those found in avocados, nuts, seeds, olive oil, and fatty seafood. These fats are essential for hormone regulation, energy production, and fat-soluble vitamin absorption.

Non-Starchy Vegetables: Add a range of non-starchy veggies, including peppers, asparagus, leafy greens, broccoli, cauliflower, and zucchini. These vegetables are high in fiber, vitamins, and minerals but low in carbohydrates.

Low-Carb Fruits: Include low-carb fruits such as berries (strawberries, blueberries, raspberries), which are lower in sugar than other fruits and include minerals and antioxidants.

Moderation in Dairy Consumption: A few Atkins Diet iterations permit small amounts of full-fat dairy products, such as cheese, butter, and cream. These offer vital fatty acids and calcium, however moderation is advised in their use.

Foods High in Fiber: Include high-fiber foods, like low-carb veggies and flaxseeds and chia seeds, to help with digestion and to help you feel fuller longer.

Portion Control: Eat in moderation to avoid overindulging in calories, especially in low-carb foods, as this might impede weight loss.

Hydration: Stay well hydrated throughout the day by drinking lots of water. This will support your body's processes and help you control your hunger.

Meal Variation: To avoid boredom and guarantee a diverse range of nutrients, strive for meal variation. To keep meals interesting, try out various recipes and ingredients.

Meal Planning: Arrange your meals ahead of time, keeping in mind the right proportions of healthy fats, low-carb veggies, and meats. Making a shopping list based on your meal plans will help you stick to your diet and resist temptations that are high in carbohydrates.

In order to support weight reduction and general health goals, creating a balanced meal plan within the Atkins Diet entails carefully choosing and combining meals rich in important nutrients while sticking to low-carb principles.

Chapter 4: DELICIOUS LOW-CARB RECIPES

Creating mouthwatering low-carb foods that fit the parameters of the Atkins Diet requires ingenuity and creativity in meal planning. It focuses on using high-protein foods as the main course of meals, such as baked fish, grilled chicken, or tofu stir-fries, as they provide vital nutrients and encourage fullness. With colorful salads, spicy vegetable meals, and creative low-carb alternatives like cauliflower rice or zucchini noodles, vegetables take center stage. These alternatives are low in carbohydrates and high in fiber, vitamins, and minerals.

Healthy fats, such as those in protein crusted with nuts or avocado, provide dishes a richer texture and essential nutrients. If you have a sweet craving, you can occasionally indulge without going against the guidelines of the diet by trying low-carb desserts made with berries or sugar substitutes. Making your own trail mix or cheese with veggies is another delicious way to have low-carb snacks in between meals.

The secret is to try new things and adjust as needed. You can get ideas from cookbooks and internet sources that are devoted to low-carb or ketogenic diets. These recipes provide a wide variety of tasty, filling, and health-conscious meals that not only fit the Atkins program's low-carb requirements but also make following the program fun and long-lasting.

Breakfasts, Lunches, and Dinners

Creating meals for breakfast, lunch, and dinner that fit the Atkins Diet guidelines requires a variety of nutrient-dense, low-carbohydrate options:

Breakfast: Choose high-protein meals such as smoothies made with protein powder and low-carb fruits, omelets stuffed with cheese and veggies, or Greek yogurt topped with berries and nuts. These choices limit carbohydrate intake while offering a full start to the day.

Lunches: Think about packing salads full of bright veggies, leafy greens, and protein sources like fish or grilled chicken for your midday meals. Other alternatives are soups made with lean meats and vegetables low in carbohydrates, or lettuce wraps stuffed with tuna or turkey. The nutrient and flavor balance of these lunches is quite pleasing.

Dinner options include a range of protein-focused dishes such as salads or non-starchy vegetables served with roasted or grilled meats (fish, poultry, or beef). Try making pizzas with cauliflower crust, stir-fries with tofu and vegetables, or zucchini noodles with pesto and grilled prawns, among other ideas. These dinner options offer a satisfying but low-carb meal.

Through meal diversification that emphasizes healthy fats, protein, and non-starchy veggies, people following the Atkins Diet can create a variety of filling and nourishing options for their meals throughout the day. These meals support weight management objectives, promote general health, and accommodate a range of tastes and dietary preferences while adhering to low-carb principles.

Snacks and Desserts

There are a number of delicious snacks and sweets that fit the low-carb guidelines within the Atkins Diet:

Snack Ideas: Try cheese and vegetable sticks, guacamole and cucumber slices, or make-your-own trail mix with almonds and seeds. These choices offer a good ratio of fiber, healthy fats, and protein to maintain steady energy levels in between meals.

Low-Carb Fruits: In moderation, savor low-carb fruits like raspberries, blueberries, and strawberries. They provide a sweet delight without causing a noticeable increase in sugar intake and are high in antioxidants.

Nuts and Seeds: Add nuts and seeds to snacks or sweets, like almonds, walnuts, chia seeds, or pumpkin seeds. They are rich in nutrients, including fiber, protein, and good fats.

Dessert Ideas: Treat yourself to low-carb treats like dark chocolate-dipped strawberries, chia seed puddings, and fruit parfaits with whipped cream. These delicacies meet your sweet tooth without going overboard on carbohydrates.

Sugar replacements: To sweeten desserts without significantly raising blood sugar levels or adding carbs, use erythritol or stevia as sugar replacements.

People can enjoy tasty treats that adhere to the Atkins Diet by choosing snacks and sweets that are high in fiber, minerals, and healthy fats while lowering their carbohydrate level. These choices promote a low-carb lifestyle and health objectives by striking a balance between satiety and enjoyment.

Simple and Flavorful Low-Carb Cooking

Within the parameters of the Atkins Diet, preparing tasty and straightforward low-carb meals requires concentrating on essential ingredients and astute cooking methods:

Embrace Protein: Begin by including foods high in protein, such as fish, eggs, lean meats, and tofu. These serve as the foundation of meals, supplying vital nutrients and encouraging satisfaction.

Healthy Fats: To give food more depth and richness, use healthy fats such avocado oil, nuts, seeds, and avocados. They contribute to a balanced diet and enhance flavors.

Non-Starchy veggies: Emphasize veggies that aren't starchy, such as bell peppers, spinach, broccoli, cauliflower, and zucchini. These vegetables are low in carbohydrates and high in color, texture, and vital nutrients.

Herbs and Spices: To enhance flavors without consuming additional carbohydrates, try experimenting with a range of herbs, spices, and seasonings. Spices like paprika or cumin, together with herbs like cilantro and basil, may elevate simple recipes.

One-Pan Meals: Make dinners on a sheet pan or skillet dishes to cut down on cooking time and effort. Mix proteins, vegetables, and seasonings in one skillet for quick, tasty dinners that need little cleaning.

Low-Carb Substitutes: Look into low-carb substitutes including lettuce wraps, zucchini noodles, and cauliflower rice. These substitutions maintain carbohydrate content while enabling the use of favorite foods.

Quick Cooking Techniques: To preserve flavors and nutrients in food while cutting down on cooking time, use quick cooking techniques like grilling, sautéing, or roasting.

Meal Prep: To make cooking easier on hectic days, think about meal planning. Meal assembly can be facilitated by preparing ingredients ahead of time.

Cooking using these techniques and experimenting with food combinations can help people create tasty, low-carb meals that fit the Atkins Diet. These techniques promote a low-carb, healthful living while enabling a wide variety of tasty dishes.

Chapter 5: EASY-TO-MAKE, LOW CARB ATKINS DIET RECIPES

LOW CARB ATKINS ATKINS DIET BREAKFAST RECIPES

Spinach and Cheese Omelette

Ingredients:

2-3 large eggs

1 cup fresh spinach, chopped

1/4 cup shredded cheddar cheese (or any cheese of your choice)

1 tablespoon olive oil or butter

Salt and pepper to taste

Instructions:

In a bowl, beat the eggs until well combined. Season with salt and pepper.

Heat olive oil or butter in a non-stick skillet over medium heat.

Add the chopped spinach to the skillet and sauté for 1-2 minutes until it wilts.

Pour the beaten eggs over the spinach in the skillet. Tilt the skillet to spread the eggs evenly.

Allow the eggs to cook for a minute or until the edges start to set.

Sprinkle the shredded cheese over one half of the omelette.

Gently fold the other half of the omelette over the cheese-covered half using a spatula.

Let it cook for an additional minute until the cheese melts and the omelette is cooked through.

Slide the omelette onto a plate and serve hot.

Avocado and Bacon Breakfast Bowl

Ingredients:

1 ripe avocado, halved and pitted

2 slices bacon

2 eggs

Salt and pepper to taste

Optional toppings: chopped fresh herbs, hot sauce, shredded cheese

Instructions:

Preheat your oven to 400°F (200°C).

Place the bacon slices on a baking sheet lined with parchment paper and bake for 10-15 minutes until crispy. Remove and set aside.

While the bacon is cooking, prepare the avocados by scooping out a little extra flesh from each half to create a larger cavity for the eggs.

Place the avocado halves in a baking dish or on a baking sheet, flesh side up.

Crack one egg into each avocado half, ensuring the yolks stay intact within the avocado cavity.

Sprinkle salt and pepper over the eggs.

Bake the avocado and eggs in the preheated oven for about 12-15 minutes, or until the eggs reach your desired level of doneness.

Remove from the oven and crumble the cooked bacon over the avocado and eggs.

Add optional toppings like fresh herbs, hot sauce, or shredded cheese if desired.

Serve immediately and enjoy your delicious avocado and bacon breakfast bowl!

Egg Tartine

Ingredients

1 ½ teaspoons extra-virgin olive oil

4 slices whole-wheat bread, lightly toasted

1 garlic clove, halved

1 medium tomato and/or avocado, sliced

4 large eggs, fried or poached

2 tablespoons herbs or microgreens

4 teaspoons capers, rinsed

Instructions

Brush oil onto toast, then rub with garlic. Top with tomato (and/or avocado) and eggs. Sprinkle with herbs (or microgreens) and capers.

Muffin-Tin Omelets with Feta & Peppers

Ingredients

Cooking spray

2 tablespoons extra-virgin olive oil

¾ cup diced onion

¼ teaspoon salt, divided

1 medium red bell pepper, diced

1 tablespoon finely chopped fresh oregano

8 large eggs

¾ cup crumbled feta cheese

½ cup low-fat milk

½ teaspoon ground pepper

2 cups chopped fresh spinach

¼ cup sliced Kalamata olives

Instructions

Preheat oven to 325 degrees F. Liberally coat a 12-cup muffin tin with cooking spray.

Heat oil in a large skillet over medium heat. Add onion and 1/8 teaspoon salt; cook, stirring, until starting to soften, about 3 minutes. Add bell pepper and oregano; cook, stirring, until the vegetables are tender and starting to brown, 4 to 5 minutes more. Remove from heat and let cool for 5 minutes.

Whisk eggs, feta, milk, pepper and the remaining 1/8 teaspoon salt in a large bowl. Stir in spinach, olives and the vegetable mixture. Divide among the prepared muffin cups.

Bake until firm to the touch, about 25 minutes. Let stand for 5 minutes before removing from the tin.

Gluten-Free Almond Flour Waffles

Ingredients

1 ½ cups almond flour

1 tablespoon granulated sugar

¾ teaspoon baking powder

¼ teaspoon baking soda

¼ teaspoon salt

2 large eggs

½ cup buttermilk

¼ cup canola oil

Directions

Preheat a waffle maker to medium heat according to manufacturer's instructions. Meanwhile, whisk almond flour, sugar, baking powder, baking soda and salt in a large bowl. Whisk eggs, buttermilk and oil in another medium bowl. Add the wet mixture to the dry mixture and stir until mostly smooth.

Lightly coat the waffle maker with cooking spray. Working in batches, add about 1/4 cup batter per waffle to the waffle maker; cook until golden brown, 5 to 7 minutes per batch. Coat the waffle maker with more cooking spray as needed between batches.

Muffin-Tin Spinach & Mushroom Mini Quiches

Ingredients

2 tablespoons extra-virgin olive oil

8 ounces fresh mixed wild mushrooms (such as oyster and shiitake), sliced

1 cup thinly sliced yellow onion

1 tablespoon minced garlic

2 teaspoons minced fresh thyme

1 (5 ounce) package fresh spinach, coarsely chopped

8 large eggs

⅔ cup whole milk

2 teaspoons Dijon mustard

½ teaspoon salt

½ teaspoon ground pepper

¾ cup shredded Gruyère cheese

Instructions

Preheat oven to 325 degrees F. Heat oil in a large nonstick skillet over medium-high heat. Add mushrooms in an even layer; cook, undisturbed, until browned on the bottom, about 4 minutes. Stir and continue to cook, stirring occasionally, until browned all over, about 5 minutes. Add onion; cook, stirring occasionally, until beginning to soften, about 4 minutes. Stir in garlic and thyme; cook, stirring, until fragrant, about 2 minutes. Add spinach; cook, stirring constantly, until just wilted, about 2 minutes. Remove from heat.

Whisk eggs, milk, Dijon, salt and pepper in a large bowl. Stir in cheese and the mushroom mixture. Coat a standard 12-cup muffin tin with cooking spray. Divide the mixture among the prepared muffin cups. Bake, uncovered, until puffed and set, about 30 minutes. Remove from the pan and serve immediately.

Easy Loaded Baked Omelet Muffins

Ingredients

3 slices bacon, chopped

2 cups finely chopped broccoli

4 scallions, sliced

8 large eggs

1 cup shredded Cheddar cheese

½ cup low-fat milk

½ teaspoon salt

½ teaspoon ground pepper

Instructions

Preheat oven to 325 degrees F. Coat a 12-cup muffin tin with cooking spray.

Cook bacon in a large skillet over medium heat until crisp, 4 to 5 minutes. Remove with a slotted spoon to a paper towel-lined plate, leaving the bacon fat in the pan. Add broccoli and scallions and cook, stirring, until soft, about 5 minutes. Remove from heat and let cool for 5 minutes.

Meanwhile, whisk eggs, cheese, milk, salt and pepper in a large bowl. Stir in the bacon and broccoli mixture. Divide the egg mixture among the prepared muffin cups.

Bake until firm to the touch, 25 to 30 minutes. Let stand for 5 minutes before removing from the muffin tin.

Avocado & Kale Omelet

Ingredients

2 large eggs

1 teaspoon low-fat milk

Pinch of salt

2 teaspoons extra-virgin olive oil, divided

1 cup chopped kale

1 tablespoon lime juice

1 tablespoon chopped fresh cilantro

1 teaspoon unsalted sunflower seeds

Pinch of crushed red pepper

Pinch of salt

¼ avocado, sliced

Instructions

Beat eggs with milk and salt in a small bowl. Heat 1 teaspoon oil in a small nonstick skillet over medium heat. Add the egg mixture and cook until the bottom is set and the center is still a bit runny, 1 to 2 minutes. Flip the omelet over and cook until set, about 30 seconds more. Transfer to a plate.

Toss kale with the remaining 1 teaspoon oil, lime juice, cilantro, sunflower seeds, crushed red pepper and a pinch of salt. Top the omelet with the kale salad and avocado.

Veggie and Cheese Frittata

Ingredients:

6 large eggs

1/2 cup chopped bell peppers (any color)

1/2 cup chopped mushrooms

1/4 cup chopped onions

1 cup baby spinach

1/2 cup shredded cheddar cheese (or any cheese of your choice)

2 tablespoons olive oil

Salt and pepper to taste

Instructions:

Preheat your oven to 350°F (175°C).

In a mixing bowl, whisk the eggs until well beaten. Season with salt and pepper.

Heat olive oil in an oven-safe skillet over medium heat.

Add the chopped onions, bell peppers, and mushrooms to the skillet. Sauté for 3-4 minutes until the vegetables soften.

Add the baby spinach to the skillet and cook for an additional 1-2 minutes until it wilts.

Spread the sautéed vegetables evenly across the skillet.

Pour the beaten eggs over the vegetables, ensuring they're evenly distributed in the skillet.

Sprinkle the shredded cheese on top of the egg and vegetable mixture.

Cook on the stovetop for 2-3 minutes until the edges start to set.

Transfer the skillet to the preheated oven and bake for 12-15 minutes or until the frittata is set and the cheese is melted and slightly golden.

Once done, remove from the oven and let it cool for a few minutes.

Slice the frittata into wedges and serve warm.

Smoked Salmon and Cream Cheese Roll-ups

Ingredients:

4 ounces smoked salmon slices

4 ounces cream cheese, softened

1 tablespoon capers (optional)

1 tablespoon chopped fresh dill

1 tablespoon lemon juice

Salt and black pepper to taste

Instructions:

In a small mixing bowl, combine the softened cream cheese, chopped dill, lemon juice, capers (if using), salt, and pepper. Mix well until thoroughly combined.

Lay out the smoked salmon slices on a clean surface.

Spread an even layer of the cream cheese mixture onto each slice of smoked salmon.

Carefully roll up each slice into a tight spiral.

Once rolled, slice the salmon rolls into smaller bite-sized pieces or leave them whole.

Arrange the smoked salmon and cream cheese roll-ups on a serving plate.

Optionally, garnish with extra dill or a sprinkle of lemon zest for added flavor.

Keto Coconut Chia Pudding

Ingredients:

1/4 cup chia seeds

1 cup unsweetened coconut milk

1/2 teaspoon vanilla extract

1 tablespoon shredded unsweetened coconut

Stevia or your preferred low-carb sweetener (optional)

Fresh berries or nuts for topping (optional)

Instructions:

In a bowl or jar, mix the chia seeds, unsweetened coconut milk, vanilla extract, and shredded coconut.

Sweeten to taste with stevia or your preferred low-carb sweetener if desired. Stir well to combine all ingredients.

Cover the bowl or jar and refrigerate it for at least 2-3 hours, or preferably overnight, to allow the chia seeds to absorb the liquid and create a pudding-like consistency.

Before serving, give the mixture a good stir. If it's too thick, you can add a splash of coconut milk to reach your desired consistency.

Divide the chia pudding into serving bowls or glasses.

Top with fresh berries or nuts for added texture and flavor if you like.

Spinach and Mushroom Crustless Quiche

Ingredients:

6 large eggs

1 cup fresh spinach, chopped

1 cup mushrooms, sliced

1/2 cup shredded cheese (cheddar, mozzarella, or your choice)

1/4 cup heavy cream or unsweetened almond milk

1 tablespoon olive oil

Salt and pepper to taste

Optional: a pinch of nutmeg or herbs of your choice

Instructions:

Preheat your oven to 350°F (175°C).

Heat olive oil in a skillet over medium heat. Add the sliced mushrooms and sauté until they release their moisture and start to brown, about 5-7 minutes. Add the chopped spinach to the skillet and cook for an additional 2-3 minutes until wilted. Set aside to cool slightly.

In a mixing bowl, whisk together the eggs, heavy cream or almond milk, salt, pepper, and optional nutmeg or herbs.

Stir in the cooked spinach and mushrooms into the egg mixture.

Grease a pie dish or baking dish with oil or cooking spray.

Pour the egg mixture into the dish and sprinkle the shredded cheese on top.

Bake in the preheated oven for 25-30 minutes or until the quiche is set in the center and the edges turn golden brown.

Remove from the oven and let it cool for a few minutes before slicing.

Peanut Butter Smoothie

Ingredients:

1 cup unsweetened almond milk or coconut milk

2 tablespoons sugar-free peanut butter or almond butter

1 scoop (about 20-25g) vanilla or chocolate-flavored low-carb protein powder

1/2 teaspoon unsweetened cocoa powder (optional)

1/2 teaspoon vanilla extract

Ice cubes (as desired for thickness)

Stevia or your preferred low-carb sweetener (optional, depending on sweetness preference)

Instructions:

In a blender, combine the almond milk (or coconut milk), sugar-free peanut butter, protein powder, cocoa powder (if using), vanilla extract, and sweetener (if desired).

Add ice cubes to the blender to achieve the desired consistency. Start with a few cubes and adjust to your preference for thickness.

Blend all the ingredients until smooth and well combined.

Taste the smoothie and adjust sweetness or thickness by adding more sweetener or ice cubes if needed.

Pour the smoothie into a glass and enjoy immediately.

Keto Veggie Breakfast Casserole

Ingredients:

6 large eggs

1 cup chopped bell peppers (mixed colors)

1 cup chopped spinach

1/2 cup chopped onions

1 cup shredded cheddar cheese

1/4 cup heavy cream

2 tablespoons olive oil

Salt and pepper to taste

Optional: cooked bacon or sausage (crumbled) for extra flavor

Instructions:

Preheat your oven to 375°F (190°C).

Heat olive oil in a skillet over medium heat. Add chopped onions and bell peppers. Sauté until softened, about 5-7 minutes. Add spinach and cook until wilted. Set aside to cool slightly.

In a mixing bowl, whisk together eggs, heavy cream, salt, and pepper until well combined.

Grease a baking dish with oil or cooking spray.

Spread the sautéed vegetables evenly on the bottom of the baking dish. If using cooked bacon or sausage, sprinkle it over the vegetables.

Pour the egg mixture over the vegetables and meat (if using), ensuring it spreads evenly.

Sprinkle shredded cheddar cheese on top.

Bake in the preheated oven for 20-25 minutes or until the eggs are set and the top is golden brown.

Once done, remove from the oven and let it cool for a few minutes before slicing.

Low-Carb Cauliflower Hash Browns

Ingredients:

2 cups grated cauliflower (about half a medium cauliflower head)

1/4 cup grated Parmesan cheese

1 large egg, beaten

1/4 teaspoon garlic powder

1/4 teaspoon onion powder

Salt and pepper to taste

Olive oil or cooking spray

Instructions:

Preheat your oven to 400°F (200°C).

Grate the cauliflower using a box grater or food processor. Place the grated cauliflower in a clean kitchen towel or cheesecloth and squeeze out excess moisture.

In a mixing bowl, combine the grated cauliflower, Parmesan cheese, beaten egg, garlic powder, onion powder, salt, and pepper. Mix well until thoroughly combined.

Line a baking sheet with parchment paper and lightly grease it with olive oil or cooking spray.

Take small handfuls of the cauliflower mixture and shape them into round patties, pressing them firmly together. Place them on the prepared baking sheet.

Bake in the preheated oven for 15-20 minutes, flipping the hash browns halfway through, until they are golden brown and crispy on the edges.

Once done, remove from the oven and let them cool for a few minutes before serving.

LOW CARB ATKINS ATKINS DIET LUNCH RECIPES

Cauliflower Crust Pizza

Ingredients:

1 medium cauliflower head

1 egg

1 cup shredded mozzarella cheese

1/4 cup grated Parmesan cheese

1 teaspoon dried oregano

1/2 teaspoon garlic powder

Salt and pepper to taste

Pizza sauce (sugar-free or low-carb)

Toppings of your choice (e.g., pepperoni, bell peppers, mushrooms, spinach)

Additional shredded mozzarella cheese (for topping)

Instructions:

Preheat your oven to 425°F (220°C). Line a baking sheet with parchment paper.

Cut the cauliflower into florets and pulse in a food processor until it resembles rice. Alternatively, you can grate the cauliflower using a box grater.

Place the riced cauliflower in a microwave-safe bowl and microwave for about 4-5 minutes. Allow it to cool for a few minutes.

Once cooled, transfer the cauliflower to a clean kitchen towel or cheesecloth and squeeze out as much moisture as possible.

In a mixing bowl, combine the squeezed cauliflower, egg, shredded mozzarella, Parmesan cheese, oregano, garlic powder, salt, and pepper. Mix until thoroughly combined.

Spread the cauliflower mixture onto the prepared baking sheet, shaping it into a round pizza crust (about 1/4 inch thick). Bake in the preheated oven for 15-20 minutes or until the crust is golden brown.

Remove the crust from the oven and let it cool slightly. Increase the oven temperature to 450°F (230°C).

Once cooled, spread pizza sauce over the crust and add your desired toppings. Sprinkle additional shredded mozzarella cheese on top.

Place the pizza back in the oven and bake for an additional 10-12 minutes or until the cheese is melted and bubbly.

Slice and serve

Zucchini Noodles with Pesto and Grilled Chicken

Ingredients:

2 medium zucchinis

2 boneless, skinless chicken breasts

1/4 cup basil pesto (store-bought or homemade)

2 tablespoons olive oil

2 cloves garlic, minced

Salt and pepper to taste

Grated Parmesan cheese for garnish (optional)

Instructions:

Using a spiralizer or vegetable peeler, create zucchini noodles ("zoodles") from the zucchinis. Set aside.

Preheat your grill or grill pan to medium-high heat.

Rub the chicken breasts with olive oil, minced garlic, salt, and pepper.

Grill the chicken for about 5-6 minutes per side or until fully cooked (reaching an internal temperature of 165°F or 74°C). Once cooked, set them aside to rest for a few minutes before slicing.

In a skillet over medium heat, add a tablespoon of olive oil. Sauté the zucchini noodles for 2-3 minutes until they are just tender but still crisp. Season with salt and pepper to taste.

Once the zucchini noodles are cooked, toss them with basil pesto until well coated.

Divide the zucchini noodles onto plates and top with sliced grilled chicken.

Garnish with grated Parmesan cheese if desired.

Lemon Garlic Shrimp with Cauliflower Rice

Ingredients:

1 pound large shrimp, peeled and deveined

3 cups cauliflower rice (store-bought or homemade)

3 tablespoons olive oil

3 cloves garlic, minced

Zest and juice of 1 lemon

2 tablespoons chopped fresh parsley

Salt and pepper to taste

Optional: Red pepper flakes for added heat

Instructions:

Heat 2 tablespoons of olive oil in a large skillet over medium heat.

Add the minced garlic to the skillet and cook for about 30 seconds until fragrant, being careful not to burn it.

Add the shrimp to the skillet and cook for 2-3 minutes per side until they turn pink and opaque. Remove the cooked shrimp from the skillet and set them aside.

In the same skillet, add the remaining tablespoon of olive oil.

Add the cauliflower rice to the skillet and sauté for 4-5 minutes until it's tender but not mushy.

Stir in the lemon zest, lemon juice, chopped parsley, salt, and pepper. Add red pepper flakes if desired for some heat.

Return the cooked shrimp to the skillet with the cauliflower rice. Toss everything together and cook for an additional minute to heat through.

Adjust seasoning to taste and serve your lemon garlic shrimp with cauliflower rice hot.

Turkey and Avocado Lettuce Wraps

Ingredients:

1 pound cooked turkey breast, sliced or shredded

1-2 avocados, sliced

8 large lettuce leaves (such as Bibb or butter lettuce)

1 tomato, sliced

1/4 red onion, thinly sliced

1/4 cup mayonnaise (look for low-carb options)

2 tablespoons Dijon mustard

Salt and pepper to taste

Optional: Sliced cucumber, bell pepper strips, or any additional veggies you enjoy

Instructions:

In a small bowl, mix together the mayonnaise and Dijon mustard to create a sauce. Set it aside.

Lay out the lettuce leaves on a clean surface.

Spread a thin layer of the mayonnaise-Dijon sauce onto each lettuce leaf.

Divide the cooked turkey breast among the lettuce leaves, placing it in the center of each leaf.

Top the turkey with avocado slices, tomato slices, red onion, and any additional veggies you'd like to add.

Season with salt and pepper to taste.

Carefully fold or roll the lettuce leaves to create wraps.

Serve your turkey and avocado lettuce wraps immediately.

Baked Salmon with Asparagus

Ingredients:

2 salmon fillets

1 bunch asparagus, trimmed

2 tablespoons olive oil

2 cloves garlic, minced

1 tablespoon lemon juice

1 teaspoon lemon zest

Salt and pepper to taste

Fresh herbs (such as dill, parsley, or thyme) for garnish

Instructions:

Preheat your oven to 400°F (200°C).

Place the salmon fillets on a baking sheet lined with parchment paper or lightly greased.

In a small bowl, mix together olive oil, minced garlic, lemon juice, lemon zest, salt, and pepper.

Brush the olive oil mixture over the salmon fillets, ensuring they are evenly coated.

Arrange the trimmed asparagus around the salmon on the baking sheet. Drizzle with a little olive oil and season with salt and pepper.

Bake in the preheated oven for 12-15 minutes or until the salmon is cooked through and flakes easily with a fork.

Remove from the oven and garnish with fresh herbs before serving.

Eggplant Parmesan with a Twist

Ingredients:

2 medium-sized eggplants, sliced into rounds

2 eggs

1 cup almond flour (or low-carb breadcrumb alternative)

1 teaspoon dried oregano

1 teaspoon dried basil

1/2 teaspoon garlic powder

Salt and pepper to taste

Olive oil for frying

2 cups sugar-free marinara sauce

2 cups shredded mozzarella cheese

Fresh basil leaves for garnish (optional)

Instructions:

Preheat your oven to 375°F (190°C).

In a shallow bowl, whisk the eggs.

In another bowl, mix together almond flour (or breadcrumbs), dried oregano, dried basil, garlic powder, salt, and pepper.

Dip each eggplant slice into the beaten eggs, then coat them in the almond flour mixture, ensuring they're evenly coated.

Heat olive oil in a skillet over medium-high heat. Fry the coated eggplant slices in batches until they're golden brown on both sides. Place them on paper towels to drain excess oil.

In a baking dish, spread a thin layer of marinara sauce. Arrange half of the fried eggplant slices over the sauce.

Top the eggplant slices with a layer of marinara sauce and sprinkle half of the shredded mozzarella cheese over it.

Add another layer of fried eggplant slices, followed by more marinara sauce and the remaining shredded mozzarella cheese.

Bake in the preheated oven for 20-25 minutes or until the cheese is melted and bubbly.

Garnish with fresh basil leaves if desired before serving.

Taco Lettuce Wraps

Ingredients:

1 pound ground beef or turkey

1 tablespoon olive oil

1 small onion, diced

2 cloves garlic, minced

1 tablespoon chili powder

1 teaspoon ground cumin

1/2 teaspoon paprika

1/4 teaspoon cayenne pepper (adjust to taste)

Salt and pepper to taste

1/2 cup sugar-free salsa

1 head iceberg or butter lettuce, leaves separated

Optional toppings: Shredded cheddar cheese, diced tomatoes, sliced avocado, sour cream (choose low-carb options)

Instructions:

Heat olive oil in a skillet over medium heat. Add diced onion and sauté until translucent.

Add minced garlic to the skillet and cook for another minute until fragrant.

Add ground beef or turkey to the skillet. Break it up with a spatula and cook until browned and cooked through.

Stir in the chili powder, ground cumin, paprika, cayenne pepper, salt, and pepper. Mix well to coat the meat evenly with the spices.

Add sugar-free salsa to the skillet and stir to combine with the meat. Cook for an additional 2-3 minutes until heated through.

Spoon the taco meat mixture onto the lettuce leaves, using them as wraps.

Add optional toppings like shredded cheddar cheese, diced tomatoes, sliced avocado, or sour cream if desired.

Chicken Caesar Salad

Ingredients:

2 boneless, skinless chicken breasts

1 tablespoon olive oil

Salt and pepper to taste

1 head romaine lettuce, chopped

1/4 cup grated Parmesan cheese

Caesar salad dressing (look for low-carb options or make your own)

Optional: Crispy bacon bits or grilled shrimp for extra protein

Instructions:

Preheat a grill or grill pan over medium-high heat.

Rub the chicken breasts with olive oil and season them with salt and pepper.

Grill the chicken for about 5-6 minutes per side or until fully cooked (reaching an internal temperature of 165°F or 74°C). Set aside to rest for a few minutes before slicing.

While the chicken is resting, prepare the salad. In a large bowl, toss the chopped romaine lettuce with grated Parmesan cheese.

Slice the grilled chicken breasts into strips.

Add the sliced chicken to the salad bowl.

Drizzle Caesar salad dressing over the salad according to your preference and toss everything together until evenly coated.

Optionally, add crispy bacon bits or grilled shrimp on top for extra flavor and protein.

Serve your Chicken Caesar Salad immediately and enjoy your Atkins-friendly lunch!

Spinach and Feta Stuffed Chicken Breast

Ingredients:

2 boneless, skinless chicken breasts

2 cups fresh spinach leaves

1/4 cup crumbled feta cheese

2 cloves garlic, minced

1 tablespoon olive oil

Salt and pepper to taste

Toothpicks or kitchen twine

Instructions:

Preheat your oven to 375°F (190°C).

In a skillet, heat olive oil over medium heat. Add minced garlic and sauté for about 30 seconds until fragrant.

Add fresh spinach leaves to the skillet and cook until wilted. Remove from heat and let it cool slightly.

Butterfly each chicken breast by slicing horizontally, but not cutting all the way through, so you can open it like a book.

Season the inside of each chicken breast with salt and pepper.

Spread half of the wilted spinach mixture onto one side of each chicken breast.

Sprinkle the crumbled feta cheese over the spinach layer.

Carefully fold the chicken breasts over the filling and secure with toothpicks or tie with kitchen twine to keep the filling inside.

Season the outside of the chicken breasts with a bit more salt and pepper.

Heat an oven-safe skillet over medium-high heat. Add a bit of olive oil.

Place the stuffed chicken breasts in the skillet and sear for about 2-3 minutes per side until browned.

Transfer the skillet to the preheated oven and bake for 20-25 minutes or until the chicken is cooked through and reaches an internal temperature of 165°F (74°C).

Remove from the oven and let the chicken rest for a few minutes before serving.

Broccoli and Cheese Soup

Ingredients:

2 cups broccoli florets

1 tablespoon olive oil

1 small onion, diced

2 cloves garlic, minced

3 cups chicken or vegetable broth

1 cup heavy cream

1 cup shredded cheddar cheese

Salt and pepper to taste

Optional: Red pepper flakes for heat, crispy bacon bits for topping

Instructions:

Heat olive oil in a pot over medium heat. Add diced onion and sauté until translucent.

Add minced garlic to the pot and cook for another minute until fragrant.

Add broccoli florets to the pot and stir for a few minutes.

Pour in the chicken or vegetable broth and bring the mixture to a boil. Reduce heat to low, cover, and simmer for about 10-15 minutes or until the broccoli is tender.

Using an immersion blender or transferring the mixture to a blender in batches, blend the soup until smooth.

Return the blended soup to the pot over low heat. Stir in the heavy cream and shredded cheddar cheese until the cheese is melted and well combined.

Season with salt and pepper to taste. Add red pepper flakes for a bit of heat if desired.

Let the soup simmer for a few more minutes until heated through.

Serve the broccoli and cheese soup hot, optionally topped with crispy bacon bits for extra flavor.

Beef and Vegetable Stir-Fry

Ingredients:

1 pound beef (flank steak or sirloin), thinly sliced

2 tablespoons soy sauce or tamari (for a gluten-free option)

2 cloves garlic, minced

1 tablespoon grated ginger

2 tablespoons olive oil

1 red bell pepper, sliced

1 green bell pepper, sliced

1 cup broccoli florets

1 cup sliced mushrooms

1 small onion, sliced

Salt and pepper to taste

Optional: Red pepper flakes for spice, sesame seeds for garnish

Instructions:

In a bowl, marinate the thinly sliced beef with soy sauce (or tamari), minced garlic, and grated ginger. Let it sit for 15-20 minutes.

Heat 1 tablespoon of olive oil in a large skillet or wok over medium-high heat.

Add the marinated beef to the skillet and stir-fry for 2-3 minutes until it's browned. Remove the beef from the skillet and set it aside.

In the same skillet, add the remaining tablespoon of olive oil.

Add sliced onions, broccoli florets, and sliced bell peppers to the skillet. Stir-fry for 3-4 minutes until the vegetables start to soften.

Add sliced mushrooms to the skillet and continue cooking for another 2-3 minutes until all the vegetables are tender-crisp.

Return the cooked beef to the skillet with the vegetables. Stir everything together and cook for an additional minute to heat through.

Season the stir-fry with salt, pepper, and red pepper flakes (if using).

Serve the beef and vegetable stir-fry hot, garnished with sesame seeds if desired.

Grilled Lemon Herb Pork Chops

Ingredients:

4 boneless pork chops

Zest and juice of 1 lemon

2 cloves garlic, minced

2 tablespoons olive oil

1 teaspoon dried thyme

1 teaspoon dried rosemary

Salt and pepper to taste

Fresh parsley for garnish (optional)

Instructions:

In a bowl, mix together the lemon zest, lemon juice, minced garlic, olive oil, dried thyme, dried rosemary, salt, and pepper to create a marinade.

Place the pork chops in a shallow dish or resealable plastic bag. Pour the marinade over the pork chops, ensuring they're evenly coated. Let them marinate in the refrigerator for at least 30 minutes or longer for better flavor.

Preheat your grill or grill pan to medium-high heat.

Remove the pork chops from the marinade and discard the excess marinade.

Grill the pork chops for about 4-5 minutes per side or until they reach an internal temperature of 145°F (63°C) for medium doneness or adjust to your preferred level of doneness.

Remove the pork chops from the grill and let them rest for a few minutes before serving.

Garnish with fresh parsley if desired and serve the grilled lemon herb pork chops hot.

Turkey and Avocado Wrap

Ingredients:

4 large lettuce leaves (such as romaine or iceberg)

8 ounces cooked turkey breast, thinly sliced

1 ripe avocado, sliced

1/2 cup cherry tomatoes, halved

1/4 cup red onion, thinly sliced

2 tablespoons mayonnaise (look for low-carb options)

1 tablespoon Dijon mustard

Salt and pepper to taste

Instructions:

Lay out the lettuce leaves on a clean surface, creating a base for your wraps.

In a small bowl, mix together the mayonnaise and Dijon mustard.

Spread the mayonnaise and mustard mixture onto each lettuce leaf.

Layer the thinly sliced turkey breast, avocado slices, cherry tomatoes, and red onion evenly among the lettuce leaves.

Season with salt and pepper to taste.

Carefully roll or fold the lettuce leaves to create wraps, securing them with toothpicks if needed.

Serve your turkey and avocado wraps immediately.

Cauliflower Fried Rice with Shrimp

Ingredients:

1 head cauliflower, grated or processed into rice-like texture

1 pound shrimp, peeled and deveined

2 tablespoons sesame oil

2 cloves garlic, minced

1/2 cup frozen peas and carrots mix

2 eggs, beaten

3 tablespoons soy sauce or tamari (for gluten-free)

2 green onions, thinly sliced

Salt and pepper to taste

Instructions:

Heat 1 tablespoon of sesame oil in a large skillet or wok over medium heat.

Add the minced garlic and cook for about 30 seconds until fragrant.

Add the shrimp to the skillet and cook for 2-3 minutes until they turn pink. Remove the shrimp and set them aside.

In the same skillet, add the remaining tablespoon of sesame oil.

Add the cauliflower rice and frozen peas and carrots mix. Stir-fry for 4-5 minutes until the vegetables are tender.

Push the cauliflower rice mixture to the side of the skillet, creating an empty space.

Pour the beaten eggs into the empty space and scramble them until cooked through.

Add the cooked shrimp back into the skillet with the cauliflower rice and veggies.

Stir in soy sauce (or tamari) and sliced green onions. Season with salt and pepper to taste.

Cook for an additional 2-3 minutes until everything is heated through.

Serve your cauliflower fried rice with shrimp hot.

Zucchini Noodle Pesto Pasta with Grilled Chicken

Ingredients:

2 medium zucchinis, spiralized into noodles

2 boneless, skinless chicken breasts

1/2 cup basil pesto (look for low-carb options or make your own)

2 tablespoons olive oil

Salt and pepper to taste

Optional: Grated Parmesan cheese for garnish

Instructions:

Preheat your grill or grill pan to medium-high heat.

Rub the chicken breasts with olive oil, salt, and pepper.

Grill the chicken for about 5-6 minutes per side or until fully cooked. Set them aside to rest for a few minutes before slicing.

In a large skillet over medium heat, add the zucchini noodles and cook for 2-3 minutes until just tender. Drain any excess moisture.

Add the basil pesto to the skillet with the zucchini noodles and toss until well coated.

Divide the pesto-coated zucchini noodles onto plates.

Slice the grilled chicken and place it on top of the zucchini noodles.

Optionally, garnish with grated Parmesan cheese before serving.

Mediterranean Chicken Salad

Ingredients:

2 boneless, skinless chicken breasts

1 tablespoon olive oil

1 teaspoon dried oregano

1 teaspoon dried basil

Salt and pepper to taste

4 cups mixed salad greens (lettuce, spinach, arugula, etc.)

1 cup cherry tomatoes, halved

1 cucumber, sliced

1/4 cup Kalamata olives, pitted and halved

1/4 cup feta cheese, crumbled

Optional: Red onion slices, chopped parsley, lemon wedges

For the Dressing:

3 tablespoons olive oil

2 tablespoons red wine vinegar

1 teaspoon Dijon mustard

1 clove garlic, minced

Salt and pepper to taste

Instructions:

Preheat your grill or grill pan to medium-high heat.

Rub the chicken breasts with olive oil and season them with dried oregano, dried basil, salt, and pepper.

Grill the chicken for about 5-6 minutes per side or until they reach an internal temperature of 165°F (74°C). Let them rest for a few minutes before slicing.

In a small bowl, whisk together the olive oil, red wine vinegar, Dijon mustard, minced garlic, salt, and pepper to make the dressing.

In a large bowl, toss the mixed salad greens, cherry tomatoes, cucumber slices, Kalamata olives, and crumbled feta cheese.

Drizzle the dressing over the salad and toss until evenly coated.

Divide the dressed salad onto plates and top each serving with sliced grilled chicken.

Optionally, add red onion slices, chopped parsley, or serve with lemon wedges on the side.

LOW CARB ATKINS ATKINS DIET DINNER RECIPES

Lemon Garlic Butter Salmon

Ingredients:

4 salmon fillets

4 tablespoons unsalted butter, melted

4 cloves garlic, minced

Zest and juice of 1 lemon

2 tablespoons chopped fresh parsley

Salt and pepper to taste

Optional: Sliced lemon for garnish

Instructions:

Preheat your oven to 375°F (190°C).

Pat dry the salmon fillets with paper towels and place them on a baking sheet lined with parchment paper or lightly greased.

In a small bowl, mix together the melted butter, minced garlic, lemon zest, lemon juice, chopped parsley, salt, and pepper.

Spoon the lemon garlic butter mixture evenly over each salmon fillet.

Place a slice of lemon on each fillet if desired.

Bake in the preheated oven for about 12-15 minutes, or until the salmon is cooked through and flakes easily with a fork.

Remove from the oven and let it rest for a minute before serving.

Low-Carb Beef and Broccoli Stir-Fry

Ingredients:

1 pound flank steak or sirloin, thinly sliced

3 cups broccoli florets

2 tablespoons olive oil

3 cloves garlic, minced

2 tablespoons soy sauce or tamari (for gluten-free)

1 tablespoon oyster sauce (look for low-carb options)

1 teaspoon sesame oil

1 teaspoon grated ginger

Salt and pepper to taste

Optional: Red pepper flakes for heat, sesame seeds for garnish

Instructions:

In a bowl, marinate the thinly sliced beef with soy sauce, oyster sauce, grated ginger, salt, and pepper. Let it sit for 15-20 minutes.

Heat 1 tablespoon of olive oil in a large skillet or wok over medium-high heat.

Add minced garlic to the skillet and cook for about 30 seconds until fragrant.

Add the marinated beef to the skillet and stir-fry for 2-3 minutes until it's browned. Remove the beef from the skillet and set it aside.

In the same skillet, add the remaining tablespoon of olive oil.

Add broccoli florets to the skillet and stir-fry for 3-4 minutes until they are tender-crisp.

Return the cooked beef to the skillet with the broccoli.

Drizzle sesame oil over the beef and broccoli mixture, and toss everything together until well combined.

Optionally, add red pepper flakes for heat if desired.

Cook for an additional 1-2 minutes to heat through.

Serve your low-carb beef and broccoli stir-fry hot, garnished with sesame seeds if desired.

Garlic Herb Butter Chicken Thighs

Ingredients:

4 bone-in, skin-on chicken thighs

4 tablespoons unsalted butter, melted

4 cloves garlic, minced

1 teaspoon dried thyme

1 teaspoon dried rosemary

Salt and pepper to taste

Fresh parsley for garnish

Instructions:

Preheat your oven to 400°F (200°C).

Pat dry the chicken thighs with paper towels and place them on a baking dish.

In a small bowl, mix together the melted butter, minced garlic, dried thyme, dried rosemary, salt, and pepper.

Brush the garlic herb butter mixture over each chicken thigh, ensuring they're evenly coated.

Bake in the preheated oven for about 35-40 minutes or until the chicken reaches an internal temperature of 165°F (74°C) and the skin is crispy and golden.

Remove from the oven and let the chicken rest for a few minutes.

Garnish with fresh parsley before serving.

Spaghetti Squash with Bolognese Sauce

Ingredients:

1 medium-sized spaghetti squash

1 pound ground beef or turkey

1 can (14 ounces) crushed tomatoes

2 cloves garlic, minced

1 onion, diced

1 carrot, grated

1 celery stalk, diced

2 tablespoons olive oil

1 teaspoon dried oregano

1 teaspoon dried basil

Salt and pepper to taste

Fresh parsley or basil for garnish

Grated Parmesan cheese (optional)

Instructions:

Preheat your oven to 375°F (190°C).

Cut the spaghetti squash in half lengthwise and scoop out the seeds. Place the squash halves on a baking sheet, cut side up.

Drizzle each half with olive oil and sprinkle with salt and pepper. Place them in the oven and bake for about 40-45 minutes until the squash is tender and the strands can be easily scraped with a fork.

While the squash is baking, prepare the Bolognese sauce. In a large skillet, heat olive oil over medium heat.

Add diced onions, minced garlic, grated carrot, and diced celery to the skillet. Cook for about 5 minutes until the vegetables are softened.

Add the ground beef or turkey to the skillet and cook until browned.

Pour in the crushed tomatoes, dried oregano, dried basil, salt, and pepper. Stir well and let it simmer for 15-20 minutes, allowing the flavors to meld.

Once the spaghetti squash is done, use a fork to scrape the flesh into strands, creating "spaghetti."

Serve the spaghetti squash topped with the Bolognese sauce.

Garnish with fresh parsley or basil. Optionally, sprinkle grated Parmesan cheese on top before serving.

Atkin Induction Friendly Crustless Quiche

Ingredients

4ounces bacon, nitrate free

1/2yellow onion, diced

6eggs

3/4cup cream, heavy

2(10 ounce) boxes spinach, thawed and drained

½lb gruyere cheese, shredded

½teaspoon salt

½teaspoon black pepper

INSTRUCTIONS

Heat oven to 350 and butter your deep pie pan or your muffin tins.

Cook bacon until crisp, drain and coarsely chop.

Use one tbsp of drippings to saute onions for 5 minutes until soft but not brown.

Combine eggs, cream, spinach, cheese, salt and pepper.

Stir in bacon and onion.

Pour mixture into prepared pan.

Bake 1 hour 15 minutes (takes about 1 hour in muffin tins).

Deviled Eggs Delight

Ingredients

4eggs, hard boiled

3pieces bacon, cooked & crumbled

2ounces cheese, shredded

2tablespoons mayonnaise

paprika (to garnish)

DIRECTIONS

Split eggs lengthwise, take out yolk.

Mix yolk with remaining ingredients except paprika.

Fill eggs with mixture and sprinkle paprika on top.

Lemon Garlic Butter Shrimp Scampi

Ingredients:

1 pound large shrimp, peeled and deveined

4 tablespoons unsalted butter

4 cloves garlic, minced

Zest and juice of 1 lemon

2 tablespoons chopped fresh parsley

Salt and pepper to taste

Optional: Red pepper flakes for heat

Instructions:

Pat dry the shrimp with paper towels and season them with salt and pepper.

In a skillet over medium heat, melt the butter.

Add minced garlic to the skillet and sauté for about 30 seconds until fragrant.

Add the shrimp to the skillet and cook for 2-3 minutes per side until they turn pink and opaque.

Stir in the lemon zest, lemon juice, chopped parsley, and red pepper flakes (if using).

Cook for an additional minute to combine the flavors and coat the shrimp evenly with the sauce.

Adjust seasoning with more salt and pepper if needed.

Serve your lemon garlic butter shrimp scampi hot, garnished with additional parsley if desired.

Stuffed Bell Peppers with Ground Turkey and Cauliflower Rice

Ingredients:

4 large bell peppers (any color), tops removed and seeds removed

1 pound ground turkey

1 cup cauliflower rice

1 small onion, finely chopped

2 cloves garlic, minced

1 can (14 ounces) diced tomatoes, drained

1 cup shredded mozzarella cheese

2 tablespoons olive oil

1 teaspoon Italian seasoning

Salt and pepper to taste

Fresh parsley for garnish

Instructions:

Preheat your oven to 375°F (190°C).

Heat olive oil in a skillet over medium heat. Add chopped onions and minced garlic. Sauté for 2-3 minutes until softened.

Add ground turkey to the skillet and cook until browned. Season with Italian seasoning, salt, and pepper.

Add cauliflower rice and drained diced tomatoes to the skillet. Cook for an additional 5-7 minutes until the cauliflower rice is tender and the mixture is well combined.

Stuff each bell pepper with the turkey and cauliflower rice mixture, pressing down gently to fill the peppers evenly.

Place the stuffed bell peppers in a baking dish. Cover the dish with aluminum foil.

Bake in the preheated oven for 25-30 minutes or until the peppers are tender.

Remove the foil, sprinkle shredded mozzarella cheese over each stuffed pepper, and return to the oven. Bake for an additional 5-7 minutes until the cheese is melted and bubbly.

Garnish with fresh parsley before serving.

Cauliflower Crust Pizza

Ingredients:

1 medium head cauliflower, riced (about 4 cups)

1 egg, beaten

1/2 cup shredded mozzarella cheese

1/4 cup grated Parmesan cheese

1 teaspoon dried oregano

1/2 teaspoon garlic powder

Salt and pepper to taste

Pizza sauce (look for low-carb options or make your own)

Toppings of your choice (such as pepperoni, bell peppers, onions, mushrooms, spinach, etc.)

Additional shredded mozzarella cheese for topping

Instructions:

Preheat your oven to 400°F (200°C). Line a baking sheet with parchment paper.

Rice the cauliflower by pulsing florets in a food processor until they resemble rice grains. Alternatively, you can use a box grater.

Place the riced cauliflower in a microwave-safe bowl and microwave for 4-5 minutes. Let it cool for a few minutes.

Transfer the cooled cauliflower rice to a clean kitchen towel or cheesecloth. Squeeze out as much moisture as possible.

In a mixing bowl, combine the cauliflower rice, beaten egg, shredded mozzarella, grated

Parmesan, dried oregano, garlic powder, salt, and pepper. Mix thoroughly.

Spread the cauliflower mixture onto the prepared baking sheet, shaping it into a round pizza crust, about 1/4 inch thick.

Bake the cauliflower crust in the preheated oven for 20-25 minutes or until it starts to turn golden brown.

Remove the crust from the oven and spread pizza sauce over it, leaving a small border for the crust.

Add your desired toppings and sprinkle additional shredded mozzarella cheese on top.

Return the pizza to the oven and bake for another 10-15 minutes or until the cheese is melted and bubbly.

Let the pizza cool for a few minutes before slicing.

Baked Lemon Herb Chicken Breasts

Ingredients:

4 boneless, skinless chicken breasts

2 tablespoons olive oil

Zest and juice of 1 lemon

2 cloves garlic, minced

1 teaspoon dried thyme

1 teaspoon dried rosemary

Salt and pepper to taste

Fresh parsley for garnish

Instructions:

Preheat your oven to 400°F (200°C).

In a small bowl, mix together the olive oil, lemon zest, lemon juice, minced garlic, dried thyme, dried rosemary, salt, and pepper to create a marinade.

Pat dry the chicken breasts with paper towels and place them in a baking dish.

Pour the marinade over the chicken breasts, ensuring they are well coated.

Let the chicken marinate for at least 20-30 minutes in the refrigerator.

Once marinated, bake the chicken in the preheated oven for 20-25 minutes or until the internal temperature reaches 165°F (74°C).

Remove the chicken from the oven and let it rest for a few minutes before serving.

Garnish with fresh parsley and serve your baked lemon herb chicken breasts.

Zucchini Lasagna

Ingredients:

4 medium zucchinis, sliced lengthwise into thin strips

1 pound ground beef or turkey

1 onion, chopped

3 cloves garlic, minced

1 can (14 ounces) crushed tomatoes

1 can (6 ounces) tomato paste

2 tablespoons olive oil

1 teaspoon dried oregano

1 teaspoon dried basil

Salt and pepper to taste

2 cups shredded mozzarella cheese

1 cup ricotta cheese

1/4 cup grated Parmesan cheese

Fresh basil for garnish (optional)

Instructions:

Preheat your oven to 375°F (190°C).

In a skillet, heat olive oil over medium heat. Add chopped onions and minced garlic. Sauté until softened.

Add ground beef or turkey to the skillet and cook until browned. Drain excess fat if necessary.

Stir in crushed tomatoes, tomato paste, dried oregano, dried basil, salt, and pepper. Simmer for 10-15 minutes.

In a separate bowl, mix together the ricotta cheese and grated Parmesan cheese.

Assemble the lasagna: In a baking dish, spread a thin layer of the meat sauce. Arrange a layer of zucchini strips over the sauce.

Spread a layer of the ricotta cheese mixture over the zucchini, followed by a layer of shredded mozzarella cheese.

Repeat the layers - sauce, zucchini, ricotta mixture, and mozzarella - until all ingredients are used, finishing with a layer of sauce and mozzarella on top.

Cover the baking dish with foil and bake in the preheated oven for 40-45 minutes.

Remove the foil and bake for an additional 10-15 minutes or until the cheese is golden and bubbly.

Let the zucchini lasagna cool for a few minutes before slicing.

Garnish with fresh basil if desired before serving.

Garlic Herb Butter Steak with Roasted Vegetables

Ingredients:

4 beef steaks (such as ribeye, sirloin, or filet mignon)

4 tablespoons unsalted butter

4 cloves garlic, minced

2 tablespoons chopped fresh parsley

1 teaspoon dried thyme

Salt and pepper to taste

1 pound mixed vegetables (such as bell peppers, zucchini, and mushrooms), cut into chunks

2 tablespoons olive oil

Optional: Fresh rosemary sprigs for garnish

Instructions:

Preheat your oven to 400°F (200°C).

Pat dry the steaks with paper towels and season them generously with salt and pepper on both sides.

In a skillet over medium-high heat, sear the steaks for 2-3 minutes on each side or until they develop a golden-brown crust. Remove from the skillet and set aside.

In the same skillet, melt the butter over medium heat. Add minced garlic, chopped parsley, dried thyme, salt, and pepper. Cook for 1-2 minutes until fragrant. Remove from heat.

Place the seared steaks on a baking sheet lined with foil or parchment paper.

Pour the garlic herb butter mixture over the steaks, ensuring they're evenly coated.

In a separate bowl, toss the mixed vegetables with olive oil, salt, and pepper.

Spread the seasoned vegetables on another baking sheet lined with foil or parchment paper.

Place both the steak and vegetables in the preheated oven. Roast the vegetables for 20-25 minutes, or until they are tender and slightly caramelized. Cook the steaks to your desired level of doneness (about 10-15 minutes for medium-rare, depending on thickness).

Remove the steak and vegetables from the oven. Let the steak rest for a few minutes before slicing.

Serve the sliced steak alongside the roasted vegetables.

Garnish with fresh rosemary sprigs if desired.

Lemon Herb Baked Cod

Ingredients:

4 cod fillets (or any white fish of your choice)

Zest and juice of 1 lemon

3 tablespoons olive oil

2 cloves garlic, minced

1 tablespoon chopped fresh parsley

1 teaspoon dried oregano

Salt and pepper to taste

Lemon slices for garnish

Optional: Thinly sliced red chili for a hint of spice

Instructions:

Preheat your oven to 375°F (190°C).

Pat dry the cod fillets with paper towels and place them in a baking dish.

In a small bowl, whisk together the lemon zest, lemon juice, olive oil, minced garlic, chopped parsley, dried oregano, salt, and pepper.

Pour the lemon herb marinade over the cod fillets, ensuring they're evenly coated. Optionally, sprinkle sliced red chili for added spice.

Let the fish marinate for about 15-20 minutes in the refrigerator.

Once marinated, place a lemon slice on each cod fillet for extra flavor.

Bake in the preheated oven for 15-20 minutes or until the fish is cooked through and flakes easily with a fork.

Serve the lemon herb baked cod hot, garnished with additional fresh parsley if desired.

Grilled Chicken Caesar Salad

Ingredients:

4 boneless, skinless chicken breasts

1 tablespoon olive oil

Salt and pepper to taste

Romaine lettuce, chopped

1/2 cup Caesar salad dressing (look for low-carb options or make your own)

1/4 cup grated Parmesan cheese

1 cup cherry tomatoes, halved

1/2 cup croutons (optional, omit for a lower-carb version)

Lemon wedges for garnish

Instructions:

Preheat your grill or grill pan to medium-high heat.

Rub the chicken breasts with olive oil and season them generously with salt and pepper.

Grill the chicken for about 5-6 minutes per side or until they reach an internal temperature of

165°F (74°C). Set them aside to rest for a few minutes before slicing.

In a large bowl, toss the chopped romaine lettuce with Caesar salad dressing until well coated.

Divide the dressed lettuce onto serving plates.

Slice the grilled chicken and place it on top of the lettuce.

Sprinkle grated Parmesan cheese over the salad.

Add cherry tomatoes and croutons (if using) as desired.

Garnish with lemon wedges for an extra citrusy kick.

Eggplant Parmesan

Ingredients:

2 large eggplants, sliced into 1/4-inch rounds

Salt

2 cups low-carb marinara sauce (look for options with fewer carbs)

2 cups shredded mozzarella cheese

1 cup grated Parmesan cheese

2 eggs

1 cup almond flour

1 teaspoon dried oregano

1 teaspoon dried basil

Olive oil for frying

Instructions:

Preheat your oven to 375°F (190°C).

Place the eggplant slices in a colander and sprinkle salt over them. Allow them to sit for about 20-30 minutes to draw out excess moisture. Rinse and pat dry with paper towels.

In a shallow bowl, whisk the eggs. In another shallow bowl, mix the almond flour, dried oregano, and dried basil.

Dip each eggplant slice into the beaten eggs, then dredge it in the almond flour mixture, coating both sides.

Heat olive oil in a large skillet over medium heat. Fry the coated eggplant slices in batches until golden brown on both sides. Place them on paper towels to drain excess oil.

In a baking dish, spread a thin layer of marinara sauce. Place a layer of fried eggplant slices on top. Add a layer of mozzarella and Parmesan cheese. Repeat the layers, finishing with a final layer of cheese on top.

Cover the baking dish with foil and bake in the preheated oven for 25-30 minutes.

Remove the foil and bake for an additional 10-15 minutes or until the cheese is golden and bubbly.

Let it cool for a few minutes before serving.

LOW CARB ATKINS ATKINS DIET DESSERT RECIPES

Keto-Friendly Chocolate Avocado Mousse

Ingredients:

2 ripe avocados

1/4 cup unsweetened cocoa powder

1/4 cup powdered erythritol or stevia (adjust to taste)

1 teaspoon vanilla extract

1/4 cup unsweetened almond milk (or any low-carb milk of choice)

Optional toppings: Unsweetened whipped cream, shaved dark chocolate, sliced almonds

Instructions:

Cut the avocados in half, remove the pits, and scoop the flesh into a blender or food processor.

Add cocoa powder, powdered erythritol or stevia, vanilla extract, and unsweetened almond milk to the blender.

Blend all the ingredients until smooth and creamy, scraping down the sides of the blender as needed.

Taste the mixture and adjust the sweetness if necessary by adding more sweetener.

Divide the chocolate avocado mousse into serving cups or bowls.

Chill in the refrigerator for at least 30 minutes to set.

Before serving, add optional toppings such as unsweetened whipped cream, shaved dark chocolate, or sliced almonds if desired.

Berry Mascarpone Parfait

Ingredients:

1 cup fresh mixed berries (such as strawberries, blueberries, raspberries)

8 ounces mascarpone cheese

1/4 cup heavy cream

2 tablespoons powdered erythritol or stevia (adjust to taste)

1 teaspoon vanilla extract

Unsweetened cocoa powder or grated dark chocolate for garnish (optional)

Instructions:

Wash and prepare the mixed berries by slicing any larger berries, if needed.

In a mixing bowl, combine the mascarpone cheese, heavy cream, powdered erythritol or stevia, and vanilla extract.

Use a hand mixer or whisk to beat the mixture until it's smooth and creamy.

In serving glasses or jars, layer the mascarpone mixture with the fresh berries, starting with a spoonful of the mascarpone mixture, then a layer of berries, and repeat until the glasses are filled.

Finish the top layer with a dollop of the mascarpone mixture and garnish with additional fresh berries.

Optionally, dust the top with a sprinkle of unsweetened cocoa powder or grated dark chocolate for decoration.

Chill the parfaits in the refrigerator for at least 30 minutes before serving.

Coconut Chia Seed Pudding

Ingredients:

1/4 cup chia seeds

1 cup unsweetened coconut milk

2 tablespoons unsweetened shredded coconut

1 tablespoon powdered erythritol or stevia (adjust to taste)

1/2 teaspoon vanilla extract

Fresh berries for topping (optional)

Instructions:

In a mixing bowl or jar, combine chia seeds, unsweetened coconut milk, shredded coconut, powdered erythritol or stevia, and vanilla extract.

Stir the mixture thoroughly until well combined. Ensure there are no clumps of chia seeds.

Cover the bowl or jar and refrigerate for at least 2-3 hours, or ideally overnight, to allow the chia seeds to absorb the liquid and create a pudding-like consistency. Stir occasionally during the initial hour to prevent clumping.

Once the chia pudding has thickened, give it a good stir to redistribute the seeds.

Serve the coconut chia seed pudding in bowls or glasses and top with fresh berries if desired.

Keto-Friendly Peanut Butter Chocolate Fat Bombs

Ingredients:

1/2 cup unsweetened creamy peanut butter

4 tablespoons coconut oil, melted

2 tablespoons unsweetened cocoa powder

2 tablespoons powdered erythritol or stevia (adjust to taste)

1/2 teaspoon vanilla extract

Pinch of salt (if the peanut butter is unsalted)

Optional: Chopped nuts or unsweetened shredded coconut for coating

Instructions:

In a mixing bowl, combine the unsweetened creamy peanut butter, melted coconut oil, unsweetened cocoa powder, powdered erythritol or stevia, vanilla extract, and a pinch of salt if using unsalted peanut butter.

Mix all the ingredients together until a smooth and well-combined mixture forms.

Place the mixture in the refrigerator for about 10-15 minutes to slightly firm up.

Once the mixture is slightly firm, roll it into small balls (about 1 inch in diameter) using your hands.

Optionally, roll the balls in chopped nuts or unsweetened shredded coconut for extra texture and flavor.

Place the fat bombs on a plate or tray lined with parchment paper and refrigerate until they are firm and set.

Lemon Cheesecake Mousse

Ingredients:

8 ounces cream cheese, softened

1/2 cup powdered erythritol or stevia (adjust to taste)

Zest and juice of 1 lemon

1 teaspoon vanilla extract

1 cup heavy whipping cream

Lemon slices or zest for garnish (optional)

Instructions:

In a mixing bowl, beat the softened cream cheese until smooth and creamy.

Add powdered erythritol or stevia, lemon zest, lemon juice, and vanilla extract to the cream cheese. Mix until well combined and smooth.

In a separate bowl, whip the heavy whipping cream until stiff peaks form.

Gently fold the whipped cream into the cream cheese mixture until fully combined. Be gentle to maintain a light and airy texture.

Divide the lemon cheesecake mousse into serving cups or dessert bowls.

Chill in the refrigerator for at least 1-2 hours to set.

Before serving, garnish with lemon slices or additional zest if desired.

Low-Carb Berry Crumble

Ingredients:

2 cups mixed berries (such as strawberries, blueberries, raspberries)

1/4 cup almond flour

1/4 cup unsweetened shredded coconut

2 tablespoons powdered erythritol or stevia (adjust to taste)

2 tablespoons butter, melted

1 teaspoon vanilla extract

Pinch of cinnamon

Optional: Chopped nuts for extra crunch

Instructions:

Preheat your oven to 350°F (175°C).

In a mixing bowl, combine the mixed berries with powdered erythritol or stevia. Toss until the berries are coated evenly.

Spread the berries evenly in a baking dish or individual ramekins.

In another bowl, mix together almond flour, unsweetened shredded coconut, melted butter, vanilla extract, a pinch of cinnamon, and optional chopped nuts until it forms a crumbly texture.

Sprinkle the crumble mixture evenly over the berries in the baking dish or ramekins.

Bake in the preheated oven for 20-25 minutes or until the crumble topping is golden brown and the berries are bubbling.

Remove from the oven and let it cool for a few minutes before serving.

Chocolate Avocado Pudding

Ingredients:

2 ripe avocados

1/4 cup unsweetened cocoa powder

1/4 cup powdered erythritol or stevia (adjust to taste)

1 teaspoon vanilla extract

Pinch of salt

Unsweetened almond milk (as needed for consistency)

Optional toppings: Fresh berries, chopped nuts, unsweetened whipped cream

Instructions:

Cut the avocados in half, remove the pits, and scoop the flesh into a blender or food processor.

Add cocoa powder, powdered erythritol or stevia, vanilla extract, and a pinch of salt to the blender.

Blend all the ingredients until smooth and creamy. If the mixture is too thick, add a splash of unsweetened almond milk to achieve the desired consistency.

Taste the pudding and adjust sweetness if necessary by adding more sweetener.

Divide the chocolate avocado pudding into serving cups or bowls.

Chill in the refrigerator for at least 30 minutes before serving.

Before serving, top with fresh berries, chopped nuts, or a dollop of unsweetened whipped cream if desired.

Coconut Flour Lemon Poppy Seed Muffins

Ingredients:

1/2 cup coconut flour

1/4 cup unsweetened shredded coconut

1/4 cup powdered erythritol or stevia (adjust to taste)

1 teaspoon baking powder

Pinch of salt

Zest of 1 lemon

3 tablespoons melted coconut oil

4 large eggs

1/4 cup unsweetened almond milk

1 tablespoon lemon juice

1 tablespoon poppy seeds

Instructions:

Preheat your oven to 350°F (175°C). Line a muffin tin with paper liners or grease the tin.

In a mixing bowl, combine the coconut flour, shredded coconut, powdered erythritol or stevia, baking powder, pinch of salt, and lemon zest.

In a separate bowl, whisk together the melted coconut oil, eggs, almond milk, and lemon juice until well combined.

Pour the wet ingredients into the dry ingredients and stir until fully combined and no lumps remain.

Fold in the poppy seeds into the batter.

Spoon the batter into the prepared muffin tin, filling each cup about 3/4 full.

Bake in the preheated oven for 18-22 minutes or until the tops are golden and a toothpick inserted into the center of a muffin comes out clean.

Remove the muffins from the oven and allow them to cool in the tin for a few minutes before transferring to a wire rack to cool completely.

Almond Butter Cookies

Ingredients:

1 cup almond butter

1/2 cup powdered erythritol or stevia (adjust to taste)

1 large egg

1 teaspoon vanilla extract

Pinch of salt

Optional: Dark chocolate chips or chopped nuts for topping

Instructions:

Preheat your oven to 350°F (175°C). Line a baking sheet with parchment paper.

In a mixing bowl, combine the almond butter, powdered erythritol or stevia, egg, vanilla extract, and a pinch of salt. Mix until well combined and a dough forms.

Scoop out tablespoon-sized portions of the dough and roll them into balls. Place them on the prepared baking sheet, leaving space between each cookie.

Flatten each cookie slightly with the back of a fork, creating a crisscross pattern on top.

Optionally, press a few dark chocolate chips or chopped nuts onto the tops of the cookies for extra flavor.

Bake in the preheated oven for 10-12 minutes or until the edges are slightly golden.

Remove the cookies from the oven and let them cool on the baking sheet for a few minutes before transferring them to a wire rack to cool completely.

Creamy Vanilla Cheesecake Bites

Ingredients:

8 ounces cream cheese, softened

1/4 cup powdered erythritol or stevia (adjust to taste)

1 large egg

1 teaspoon vanilla extract

Optional: Sugar-free fruit preserves or berries for topping

Instructions:

Preheat your oven to 325°F (163°C). Line a mini muffin tin with paper liners.

In a mixing bowl, beat the softened cream cheese until smooth and creamy.

Add powdered erythritol or stevia, egg, and vanilla extract to the cream cheese. Mix until well combined and smooth.

Spoon the cheesecake mixture into the mini muffin tin, filling each cup almost to the top.

Optional: Add a small dollop of sugar-free fruit preserves or place a berry on top of each cheesecake bite.

Bake in the preheated oven for 12-15 minutes or until the edges are set but the centers are slightly jiggly.

Remove the cheesecake bites from the oven and allow them to cool in the tin for a few minutes before transferring them to a wire rack to cool completely.

Once cooled, chill the cheesecake bites in the refrigerator for at least an hour before serving.

Chocolate Avocado Truffles

Ingredients:

2 ripe avocados

1/4 cup unsweetened cocoa powder

1/4 cup powdered erythritol or stevia (adjust to taste)

1 teaspoon vanilla extract

Pinch of salt

Unsweetened shredded coconut or cocoa powder for coating

Instructions:

Cut the avocados in half, remove the pits, and scoop the flesh into a mixing bowl.

Add cocoa powder, powdered erythritol or stevia, vanilla extract, and a pinch of salt to the bowl.

Mash and mix all the ingredients together until well combined and smooth.

Place the mixture in the refrigerator for about 30 minutes to firm up slightly.

Once the mixture is firm enough to handle, scoop out tablespoon-sized portions and roll them into balls.

Roll each ball in unsweetened shredded coconut or cocoa powder to coat evenly.

Place the coated truffles on a plate or tray lined with parchment paper.

Chill the truffles in the refrigerator for at least 1 hour before serving.

Peanut Butter Chocolate Fat Bombs

Ingredients:

1/2 cup unsweetened creamy peanut butter

4 tablespoons coconut oil, melted

2 tablespoons unsweetened cocoa powder

2 tablespoons powdered erythritol or stevia (adjust to taste)

1/2 teaspoon vanilla extract

Pinch of salt (if the peanut butter is unsalted)

Optional: Chopped nuts or unsweetened shredded coconut for topping

Instructions:

In a mixing bowl, combine the unsweetened creamy peanut butter, melted coconut oil, unsweetened cocoa powder, powdered erythritol or stevia, vanilla extract, and a pinch of salt if using unsalted peanut butter.

Mix all the ingredients together until well combined and smooth.

Line a mini muffin tin with paper liners.

Spoon the peanut butter mixture into each mini muffin cup, filling them about halfway.

Optionally, sprinkle chopped nuts or unsweetened shredded coconut on top of each fat bomb for added texture.

Place the muffin tin in the freezer and let the fat bombs set for at least 30 minutes, or until firm.

Once set, remove the fat bombs from the muffin tin and store them in an airtight container in the freezer.

Keto Lemon Bars

Crust Ingredients:

1 cup almond flour

1/4 cup powdered erythritol or stevia (adjust to taste)

4 tablespoons melted butter

Filling Ingredients:

4 large eggs

1 cup powdered erythritol or stevia (adjust to taste)

Zest and juice of 2 lemons

2 tablespoons almond flour

1/2 teaspoon baking powder

Optional: Powdered erythritol for dusting (after baking)

Instructions:

Preheat your oven to 350°F (175°C). Line an 8x8-inch baking dish with parchment paper, leaving some overhang for easy removal.

In a mixing bowl, combine the almond flour, powdered erythritol or stevia, and melted butter for the crust. Mix until well combined.

Press the crust mixture evenly into the bottom of the prepared baking dish. Bake for 10-12 minutes or until lightly golden. Remove from the oven and set aside.

In another bowl, whisk together the eggs, powdered erythritol or stevia, lemon zest, and lemon juice until well combined.

Add the almond flour and baking powder to the egg mixture and whisk until smooth.

Pour the lemon filling over the baked crust.

Bake for an additional 20-25 minutes or until the filling is set.

Allow the bars to cool completely in the baking dish.

Once cooled, lift the parchment paper to remove the bars from the dish. Dust the top with powdered erythritol if desired.

Cut into squares and refrigerate before serving.

Keto Chocolate Mousse

Ingredients:

1 cup heavy whipping cream

2 tablespoons unsweetened cocoa powder

2 tablespoons powdered erythritol or stevia (adjust to taste)

1 teaspoon vanilla extract

Optional: Unsweetened chocolate shavings for garnish

Instructions:

Chill a mixing bowl in the freezer for about 10-15 minutes before starting.

In the chilled mixing bowl, pour in the heavy whipping cream.

Using a hand mixer or stand mixer, whip the cream until it thickens and reaches soft peaks.

Add unsweetened cocoa powder, powdered erythritol or stevia, and vanilla extract to the whipped cream.

Continue to whip the mixture until it forms stiff peaks and becomes a mousse-like consistency.

Taste and adjust the sweetness if needed by adding more powdered erythritol or stevia.

Spoon the chocolate mousse into serving bowls or glasses.

Optionally, garnish with unsweetened chocolate shavings.

Chill the mousse in the refrigerator for at least 30 minutes before serving.

Keto-Friendly Berry Chia Seed Pudding

Ingredients:

1 cup unsweetened almond milk (or any low-carb milk of choice)

1/4 cup chia seeds

2 tablespoons powdered erythritol or stevia (adjust to taste)

1 teaspoon vanilla extract

1 cup mixed berries (such as strawberries, blueberries, raspberries)

Optional: Unsweetened shredded coconut for topping

Instructions:

In a mixing bowl, combine the unsweetened almond milk, chia seeds, powdered erythritol or stevia, and vanilla extract. Stir well to combine.

Let the mixture sit for about 5 minutes, then stir again to prevent clumping. Repeat this process a couple of times over 15-20 minutes until the chia seeds begin to absorb the liquid and the mixture thickens.

Once the pudding reaches a pudding-like consistency, divide it into serving cups or bowls.

Top the chia seed pudding with mixed berries.

Optionally, sprinkle some unsweetened shredded coconut over the top for added texture and flavor.

Chill the pudding in the refrigerator for at least 1-2 hours or until completely set.

LOW CARB ATKINS ATKINS DIET SOUP RECIPES

Creamy Broccoli Cheddar Soup

Ingredients:

4 cups fresh broccoli florets

1 tablespoon olive oil

1 small onion, diced

2 cloves garlic, minced

4 cups chicken or vegetable broth

1 cup heavy cream

2 cups shredded cheddar cheese

Salt and pepper to taste

Optional: Crispy bacon bits for garnish

Instructions:

In a large pot, heat olive oil over medium heat. Add diced onion and garlic, sauté until translucent and fragrant.

Add broccoli florets to the pot and sauté for a few minutes.

Pour in the chicken or vegetable broth, covering the broccoli. Bring to a simmer and cook until the broccoli is tender, about 10-12 minutes.

Use an immersion blender or transfer the mixture to a blender to puree until smooth. Be cautious when blending hot liquids.

Return the pureed mixture to the pot over low heat. Stir in the heavy cream and shredded cheddar cheese, allowing the cheese to melt into the soup.

Season with salt and pepper to taste. Adjust consistency with more broth if desired.

Simmer the soup for a few more minutes until it reaches your desired thickness.

Serve the soup hot, garnished with crispy bacon bits if desired.

Roasted Tomato Basil Soup

Ingredients:

8-10 medium-sized tomatoes, halved

1 onion, roughly chopped

4 cloves garlic, minced

2 tablespoons olive oil

4 cups chicken or vegetable broth

1/2 cup fresh basil leaves, chopped

Salt and pepper to taste

Optional: Heavy cream or coconut cream for garnish

Instructions:

Preheat your oven to 400°F (200°C).

Place the halved tomatoes, chopped onion, and minced garlic on a baking sheet. Drizzle with olive oil and season with salt and pepper.

Roast the tomato mixture in the preheated oven for 25-30 minutes or until the tomatoes are slightly charred and softened.

Transfer the roasted tomatoes, onions, and garlic to a large pot. Add the chicken or vegetable broth.

Bring the mixture to a boil, then reduce heat and let it simmer for about 15-20 minutes to allow the flavors to meld together.

Use an immersion blender or transfer the mixture to a blender to puree until smooth.

Return the soup to the pot over low heat. Stir in the chopped fresh basil leaves.

Taste and adjust seasoning with salt and pepper as needed.

Serve the soup hot, optionally garnished with a drizzle of heavy cream or coconut cream for added richness.

Creamy Cauliflower Soup

Ingredients:

1 head cauliflower, chopped into florets

1 onion, chopped

2 cloves garlic, minced

4 cups chicken or vegetable broth

1 cup heavy cream

2 tablespoons olive oil

Salt and pepper to taste

Optional: Crispy bacon bits or grated cheddar cheese for garnish

Instructions:

In a large pot, heat olive oil over medium heat. Add chopped onion and garlic, sauté until softened and fragrant.

Add cauliflower florets to the pot and sauté for a few minutes.

Pour in the chicken or vegetable broth, covering the cauliflower. Bring to a boil, then reduce heat and simmer until the cauliflower is tender, about 15-20 minutes.

Use an immersion blender or transfer the mixture to a blender to puree until smooth.

Return the pureed mixture to the pot over low heat. Stir in the heavy cream, allowing it to simmer for an additional 5-10 minutes.

Season with salt and pepper to taste.

Serve the soup hot, garnished with crispy bacon bits or grated cheddar cheese if desired.

Zucchini and Basil Soup

Ingredients:

4 medium zucchinis, sliced

1 onion, chopped

2 cloves garlic, minced

4 cups vegetable or chicken broth

1/2 cup fresh basil leaves, chopped

2 tablespoons olive oil

Salt and pepper to taste

Optional: Grated Parmesan cheese for garnish

Instructions:

In a large pot, heat olive oil over medium heat. Add chopped onion and minced garlic, sauté until softened and fragrant.

Add sliced zucchinis to the pot and sauté for a few minutes until they begin to soften.

Pour in the vegetable or chicken broth, covering the zucchinis. Bring to a boil, then reduce heat and simmer for about 15-20 minutes until the zucchinis are tender.

Use an immersion blender or transfer the mixture to a blender to puree until smooth.

Return the pureed soup to the pot over low heat. Stir in the chopped fresh basil leaves.

Season with salt and pepper to taste.

Serve the soup hot, optionally garnished with grated Parmesan cheese for added flavor.

Spinach and Mushroom Soup

Ingredients:

8 oz fresh mushrooms, sliced

4 cups fresh spinach leaves

1 onion, chopped

2 cloves garlic, minced

4 cups vegetable or chicken broth

2 tablespoons olive oil

Salt and pepper to taste

Optional: Heavy cream or grated Parmesan cheese for garnish

Instructions:

In a large pot, heat olive oil over medium heat. Add chopped onion and minced garlic, sauté until softened and fragrant.

Add sliced mushrooms to the pot and sauté until they begin to release their juices.

Pour in the vegetable or chicken broth, covering the mushrooms. Bring to a boil, then reduce heat and let it simmer for about 10-12 minutes.

Add fresh spinach leaves to the pot and cook for an additional 3-5 minutes until the spinach wilts.

Use an immersion blender or transfer the mixture to a blender to puree about half of the soup, leaving some chunks for texture.

Return the soup to the pot over low heat. Season with salt and pepper to taste.

Serve the soup hot, optionally garnished with a drizzle of heavy cream or grated Parmesan cheese for added richness.

Creamy Asparagus Soup

Ingredients:

1 lb asparagus, tough ends trimmed and chopped

1 onion, chopped

2 cloves garlic, minced

4 cups vegetable or chicken broth

1/2 cup heavy cream

2 tablespoons olive oil

Salt and pepper to taste

Optional: Lemon zest or fresh herbs for garnish

Instructions:

In a large pot, heat olive oil over medium heat. Add chopped onion and minced garlic, sauté until translucent and fragrant.

Add the chopped asparagus to the pot and sauté for a few minutes until slightly softened.

Pour in the vegetable or chicken broth, covering the asparagus. Bring to a boil, then reduce heat and simmer for about 15-20 minutes or until the asparagus is tender.

Use an immersion blender or transfer the mixture to a blender to puree until smooth.

Return the pureed soup to the pot over low heat. Stir in the heavy cream, allowing it to simmer for an additional 5-10 minutes.

Season with salt and pepper to taste.

Serve the soup hot, optionally garnished with a sprinkle of lemon zest or fresh herbs for added brightness.

Curry Chicken Cauliflower Soup

Ingredients:

1 lb boneless, skinless chicken breasts, diced

1 head cauliflower, chopped into florets

1 onion, chopped

2 cloves garlic, minced

1 can (14 oz) coconut milk

4 cups chicken broth

2 tablespoons curry powder

2 tablespoons olive oil

Salt and pepper to taste

Fresh cilantro for garnish (optional)

Instructions:

In a large pot, heat olive oil over medium heat. Add diced chicken and sauté until lightly browned. Remove the chicken from the pot and set aside.

In the same pot, add chopped onion and minced garlic. Sauté until onions are translucent.

Add cauliflower florets to the pot and sauté for a few minutes.

Sprinkle curry powder over the vegetables and stir to coat evenly.

Pour in the chicken broth and coconut milk, then add the browned chicken back into the pot.

Bring the mixture to a gentle boil, then reduce heat and let it simmer for about 15-20 minutes until the cauliflower is tender.

Use an immersion blender or transfer the mixture to a blender to puree until smooth.

Season with salt and pepper to taste.

Serve the soup hot, optionally garnished with fresh cilantro for an extra burst of flavor.

Creamy Roasted Red Pepper Soup

Ingredients:

3 large red bell peppers

1 onion, chopped

2 cloves garlic, minced

4 cups vegetable or chicken broth

1/2 cup heavy cream

2 tablespoons olive oil

Salt and pepper to taste

Optional: Smoked paprika or fresh herbs for garnish

Instructions:

Preheat your oven to broil. Place whole red bell peppers on a baking sheet and roast them in the oven, turning occasionally, until the skins are charred and blistered. This usually takes about 15-20 minutes. Remove from the oven and let them cool.

Once cooled, peel off the charred skin from the roasted red peppers, remove the seeds, and roughly chop the flesh.

In a large pot, heat olive oil over medium heat. Add chopped onion and minced garlic, sauté until translucent and fragrant.

Add the chopped roasted red peppers to the pot and sauté for a few minutes.

Pour in the vegetable or chicken broth, covering the peppers and onions. Bring to a boil, then reduce heat and simmer for about 10-15 minutes.

Use an immersion blender or transfer the mixture to a blender to puree until smooth.

Return the pureed soup to the pot over low heat. Stir in the heavy cream, allowing it to simmer for an additional 5-10 minutes.

Season with salt and pepper to taste.

Serve the soup hot, optionally garnished with a sprinkle of smoked paprika or fresh herbs for added flavor.

Italian Sausage and Spinach Soup

Ingredients:

1 lb Italian sausage, casings removed

1 onion, chopped

2 cloves garlic, minced

4 cups chicken or beef broth

1 can (14 oz) diced tomatoes

4 cups fresh spinach leaves

1 teaspoon Italian seasoning

Salt and pepper to taste

Grated Parmesan cheese for garnish (optional)

Instructions:

In a large pot, cook the Italian sausage over medium heat, breaking it into crumbles with a spoon, until browned and cooked through. Remove any excess grease if needed.

Add chopped onion to the pot and sauté until translucent. Add minced garlic and cook for another minute.

Pour in the chicken or beef broth, diced tomatoes (with their juices), and Italian seasoning. Bring the mixture to a boil.

Reduce heat to a simmer and let it cook for about 10-15 minutes to allow the flavors to meld together.

Stir in the fresh spinach leaves and continue simmering for an additional 5 minutes until the spinach wilts.

Season with salt and pepper to taste.

Serve the soup hot, optionally garnished with grated Parmesan cheese for added flavor.

Creamy Chicken and Mushroom Soup

Ingredients:

1 lb boneless, skinless chicken thighs, diced

8 oz mushrooms, sliced

1 onion, chopped

2 cloves garlic, minced

4 cups chicken broth

1 cup heavy cream

2 tablespoons butter

2 tablespoons olive oil

Salt and pepper to taste

Fresh parsley for garnish (optional)

Instructions:

In a large pot, heat olive oil over medium heat. Add diced chicken thighs and cook until browned. Remove the chicken from the pot and set aside.

Add butter to the pot and sauté chopped onion and minced garlic until softened and fragrant.

Add sliced mushrooms to the pot and cook until they release their moisture and start to brown.

Return the cooked chicken to the pot and pour in the chicken broth. Bring to a boil, then reduce heat and let it simmer for about 10-15 minutes.

Stir in the heavy cream and let the soup simmer for an additional 5-10 minutes.

Season with salt and pepper to taste.

Serve the soup hot, garnished with fresh parsley if desired.

Spicy Cauliflower and Cheddar Soup

Ingredients:

1 head cauliflower, chopped into florets

1 onion, diced

2 cloves garlic, minced

4 cups vegetable or chicken broth

1 cup sharp cheddar cheese, shredded

1/2 cup heavy cream

2 tablespoons olive oil

1 teaspoon paprika

1/2 teaspoon cayenne pepper (adjust to taste)

Salt and pepper to taste

Optional: Chopped green onions for garnish

Instructions:

In a large pot, heat olive oil over medium heat. Add diced onion and minced garlic, sauté until onions are translucent.

Add cauliflower florets to the pot and sauté for a few minutes.

Pour in the vegetable or chicken broth, covering the cauliflower. Bring to a boil, then reduce heat and simmer for about 15-20 minutes or until the cauliflower is tender.

Use an immersion blender or transfer the mixture to a blender to puree until smooth.

Return the pureed soup to the pot over low heat. Stir in the heavy cream, shredded cheddar cheese, paprika, and cayenne pepper.

Let the soup simmer for an additional 5-10 minutes, stirring occasionally until the cheese melts and the soup thickens.

Season with salt and pepper to taste.

Serve the soup hot, garnished with chopped green onions if desired.

Turkey and Vegetable Soup

Ingredients:

1 lb ground turkey

1 onion, chopped

2 carrots, diced

2 celery stalks, diced

2 cloves garlic, minced

4 cups chicken or vegetable broth

1 can (14 oz) diced tomatoes

1 teaspoon dried thyme

1 teaspoon dried oregano

Salt and pepper to taste

Fresh parsley for garnish (optional)

Instructions:

In a large pot, cook the ground turkey over medium heat until browned. Drain any excess fat and set aside.

In the same pot, add chopped onion, diced carrots, diced celery, and minced garlic. Sauté until the vegetables are tender.

Add the cooked turkey back to the pot along with the chicken or vegetable broth, diced tomatoes (with their juices), dried thyme, and dried oregano.

Bring the mixture to a boil, then reduce heat and simmer for about 15-20 minutes to allow the flavors to blend.

Season with salt and pepper to taste.

Serve the soup hot, garnished with fresh parsley if desired.

Creamy Broccoli and Cheese Soup

Ingredients:

4 cups fresh broccoli florets

1 onion, chopped

2 cloves garlic, minced

4 cups chicken or vegetable broth

1 cup heavy cream

2 cups shredded cheddar cheese

2 tablespoons butter

Salt and pepper to taste

Optional: Crispy bacon bits for garnish

Instructions:

In a large pot, melt butter over medium heat. Add chopped onion and minced garlic, sauté until softened and fragrant.

Add broccoli florets to the pot and sauté for a few minutes until they begin to soften.

Pour in the chicken or vegetable broth, covering the broccoli. Bring to a boil, then reduce heat and simmer for about 10-15 minutes until the broccoli is tender.

Use an immersion blender or transfer the mixture to a blender to puree until smooth.

Return the pureed soup to the pot over low heat. Stir in the heavy cream and shredded cheddar cheese, allowing the cheese to melt into the soup.

Season with salt and pepper to taste.

Serve the soup hot, optionally garnished with crispy bacon bits for added flavor.

Mexican Chicken and Cauliflower Rice Soup

Ingredients:

1 lb boneless, skinless chicken breasts, diced

1 onion, chopped

2 cloves garlic, minced

4 cups chicken broth

1 can (14 oz) diced tomatoes with green chilies

2 cups cauliflower rice

1 teaspoon cumin

1 teaspoon chili powder

Salt and pepper to taste

Fresh cilantro for garnish (optional)

Lime wedges for serving (optional)

Instructions:

In a large pot, heat a bit of oil over medium heat.
Add diced chicken and cook until browned and

cooked through. Remove from the pot and set aside.

In the same pot, add chopped onion and sauté until translucent. Add minced garlic and cook for another minute.

Pour in the chicken broth, diced tomatoes with green chilies (undrained), and cauliflower rice. Bring to a simmer.

Stir in the cooked chicken, cumin, and chili powder. Simmer for about 15-20 minutes.

Season with salt and pepper to taste.

Serve the soup hot, garnished with fresh cilantro and a lime wedge if desired.

Creamy Spinach and Artichoke Soup

Ingredients:

2 cups fresh spinach leaves, chopped

1 can (14 oz) artichoke hearts, drained and chopped

1 onion, chopped

2 cloves garlic, minced

4 cups chicken or vegetable broth

1 cup heavy cream

1 cup shredded mozzarella cheese

2 tablespoons butter

Salt and pepper to taste

Optional: Grated Parmesan cheese for garnish

Instructions:

In a large pot, melt butter over medium heat. Add chopped onion and minced garlic, sauté until softened and fragrant.

Add chopped spinach and chopped artichoke hearts to the pot. Cook for a few minutes until spinach wilts.

Pour in the chicken or vegetable broth and bring to a simmer. Let it cook for about 10-15 minutes.

Stir in the heavy cream and shredded mozzarella cheese, allowing the cheese to melt into the soup.

Continue to simmer for an additional 5-10 minutes, stirring occasionally.

Season with salt and pepper to taste.

Serve the soup hot, optionally garnished with grated Parmesan cheese for added flavor.

Creamy Tomato Basil Soup

Ingredients:

4 cups fresh tomatoes, chopped

1 onion, chopped

2 cloves garlic, minced

4 cups vegetable or chicken broth

1/2 cup heavy cream

1/4 cup fresh basil leaves, chopped

2 tablespoons olive oil

Salt and pepper to taste

Optional: Fresh basil leaves for garnish

Instructions:

In a large pot, heat olive oil over medium heat. Add chopped onion and minced garlic, sauté until onions are translucent.

Add chopped tomatoes to the pot and cook for about 5-7 minutes until they begin to soften.

Pour in the vegetable or chicken broth, covering the tomatoes and onions. Bring to a boil, then reduce heat and simmer for about 15-20 minutes.

Use an immersion blender or transfer the mixture to a blender to puree until smooth.

Return the pureed soup to the pot over low heat. Stir in the heavy cream and chopped fresh basil.

Season with salt and pepper to taste.

Simmer the soup for an additional 5-10 minutes, allowing the flavors to meld together.

Serve the soup hot, optionally garnished with fresh basil leaves.

Chapter 5: FITNESS AND EXERCISE ON ATKINS

For overall health and wellness, incorporating exercise and fitness into the Atkins Diet plan is essential. The method, which includes a variety of activities like aerobic workouts, strength training, and flexibility routines, promotes regular physical activity. The focus is on adding at least 150 minutes a week of moderate-intensity aerobic activity to a regimen of strength training to develop muscle and flexibility exercises to improve mobility and prevent injuries.

Customizing the workout program to each person's fitness level, preferences, and medical circumstances is essential. In order to achieve long-term adherence and benefits, consistency is emphasized and the creation of a routine that matches one's lifestyle is encouraged. Additionally taken into account are hydration and post-workout nutrition, with a focus on the significance of maintaining hydration and having a well-balanced meal or snack after exercise for the best possible recovery.

Prioritizing safety, it is advised that before beginning a new workout regimen, individuals with pre-existing health difficulties in particular should speak with fitness experts or healthcare specialists. People can attain holistic wellness, supporting weight management, cardiovascular health, muscle strength, and general well-being within the Atkins lifestyle, by combining the dietary principles of the Atkins Diet with regular physical activity.

Role of Exercise in Atkins

Exercise enhances general health and maximizes the benefits of the Atkins Diet, making it a valuable addition to the diet:

Enhanced Weight Management: By promoting fat loss and calorie burning, exercise in conjunction with the Atkins Diet can help with weight management. It enhances the weight reduction process by balancing the diet's emphasis on rerouting the body's fuel supply to stored fat.

Enhanced Metabolic Health: Insulin sensitivity and blood sugar management are two metabolic health indicators that can be enhanced by physical activity. Exercise has the potential to augment the metabolic advantages of the Atkins Diet when combined with its low-carb principles.

Strength and Muscle Health: Exercise, especially strength training, contributes to the maintenance and growth of muscle mass. This is particularly crucial to make sure that the body loses fat instead of muscle during weight loss.

Improved Fitness Levels: Consistent exercise, whether it be strength- or aerobic-based, raises one's physical capabilities, endurance, and level of fitness. When combined with the Atkins Diet's dietary modifications, it promotes general health and wellbeing.

Mental Health: Studies have shown that exercise has a beneficial effect on mental health by lowering stress and elevating mood. This psychological advantage can support the general health and well-being that the Atkins Diet emphasizes.

Long-Term Health: Engaging in regular physical activity lowers the chance of developing a number of chronic illnesses, including diabetes, heart disease, and some types of cancer. Long-term health objectives are supported when the Atkins Diet is combined with exercise.

Personalized Approach: Adapting the workout regimen to each person's interests and degree of fitness guarantees that it enhances and prolongs the benefits of the Atkins Diet.

People can maximize their weight loss efforts, enhance overall health markers, and attain a more comprehensive approach to health and wellbeing within the Atkins lifestyle by realizing the significance of exercise as a complementing component of the diet.

Fitness Routines for Success

Creating effective exercise regimens within the parameters of the Atkins Diet requires careful preparation and commitment:

Routine Development: Make an organized workout schedule that includes a variety of activities, including flexibility, strength, and cardiovascular conditioning. Create a timetable that works for your objectives and way of life.

Gradual Progression: As fitness increases, start at a comfortable level and progressively up the volume, duration, or frequency of workouts. This step-by-step method keeps people safe and promotes consistent advancement.

Diversification: Use a range of workouts to work out various muscle groups and avoid boredom. For a well-rounded routine, switch up your aerobic, resistance, and flexibility routines.

Consistency: Make a commitment to consistent activity, with a weekly goal of at least 150 minutes of moderate-intense aerobic exercise in addition to strength training sessions. Maintaining consistency is essential for long-term gains.

Balanced Approach: To increase general fitness, strike a balance between strength and cardio training. Strength training maintains muscle mass and increases metabolism, whilst cardio activities enhance cardiovascular health and burn calories.

Adaptation: Allow yourself to be adaptable and change your routine to suit evolving needs or tastes. To keep the program interesting and productive, try new activities, mix up the workouts, or make other adjustments.

Rest and Recovery: To avoid burnout and promote muscle repair, give yourself enough time to rest and recover in between workouts. Observe your body and refrain from overtraining.

Monitoring Development: Observe exercises, advancement, and objectives. Tracking gains in strength, weight, or fitness levels can inspire you and help you modify the program as necessary.

Nutrition and Hydration: Eat right and stay hydrated to support your exercise regimen. Sufficient protein consumption on the Atkins Diet facilitates the repair of muscles, and maintaining proper hydration is crucial for peak performance.

Combining Exercise and Low-Carb Eating

Exercise and a low-carb diet, like the Atkins Diet, work in concert to provide a potent synergy that enhances general health and wellbeing:

Enhanced Weight Loss: By motivating the body to burn fat that has been stored as fuel, a low-carb diet and exercise regimen help people lose weight. Exercise increases fat metabolism and calorie burning, which is a beneficial addition to a low-carb diet.

Enhanced Energy Use: Exercise and a low-carb diet combine to maximize utilisation of energy. The body uses stored fat more effectively and gains endurance during exercises when it isn't as dependent on carbs.

Muscle Preservation: Frequent physical activity, particularly strength training, aids in the maintenance and growth of muscle mass. This ensures that weight loss predominantly targets fat storage rather than muscle tissue, which is a complement to the low-carb approach.

Metabolic Health: Insulin sensitivity, blood sugar management, and lipid profiles are all improved when low-carbohydrate diet and exercise are coupled. Synergistic effects on overall metabolic health parameters may be observed with this combination.

Enhanced Fitness: Exercise increases strength, flexibility, and cardiovascular fitness, which is a compliment to the Atkins Diet. This combination improves physical capacities and promotes a healthy lifestyle in general.

Sustainable Weight management: By encouraging calorie restriction, fat utilization, and an improved body composition, exercise and a low-carb diet plan help sustainable weight management.

Personalized Approach: Effectiveness and long-term adherence are ensured by customizing the low-carb diet and exercise regimen to each person's preferences, fitness level, and health objectives.

Drinking enough water and eating a balanced diet consisting mostly of low-carb meals as suggested by the Atkins Diet will help you perform better during exercise, recover from it, and feel better overall.

Through the combination of exercise and low-carb diet, people can increase their general fitness levels, aid weight reduction, optimize metabolic health, and achieve complete health improvements while adhering to the Atkins lifestyle.

Chapter 6: LONG-TERM WELLNESS WITH ATKINS

The Atkins Diet is a lifestyle strategy focused on long-term wellness, not just weight loss. By highlighting whole, nutrient-dense foods including lean proteins, healthy fats, and non-starchy veggies, it encourages long-lasting improvements in eating patterns. It emphasizes weight management techniques that help sustain a healthy weight over time, going beyond initial weight loss. The goal of the diet is to improve metabolic health markers by restricting refined carbohydrates and sugars. This will lower the risk of chronic illnesses and contribute to general wellness.

Incorporating exercise is recommended to boost the benefits of the diet by promoting physical fitness, maintaining muscle mass, and improving metabolic advantages. Flexibility in the diet promotes long-term adherence and sustainability as a lifestyle choice by enabling adaptability to personal tastes and health demands. Beyond weight and metabolic health, the diet may also have positive effects on energy levels, mood stability, and inflammation reduction, all of which can contribute to a person's overall sense of wellbeing.

If you want to follow the Atkins Diet for the long term, you have to keep learning and adjusting to make it more effective. This lifestyle choice seeks to achieve long-term, comprehensive well-being, which includes weight control, improved health markers, increased vigor, and a holistic sense of wellness, rather than just quick fixes.

Maintaining Weight Loss and Health Benefits

Important tactics for long-term success are needed to maintain the weight loss and health advantages of the Atkins Diet:

Adherence to the Atkins Diet: Make the diet a long-term way of life rather than a temporary fix. Accept its recommendations for a balanced diet that prioritizes whole foods in order to maintain weight loss and overall health gains.

Moderation and Portion Control: Even while eating low-carb foods, control your calorie intake by eating in moderation. Eat in moderation to avoid overindulging and to help you maintain your weight.

Frequent Physical Activity: As part of your lifestyle, keep up your regular exercise regimen. Maintaining muscle mass and managing weight are two benefits of physical activity that contribute to overall health.

Eat with awareness: Pay attention to the foods you choose and the way you eat. Pay attention to your body's signals of hunger and fullness while choosing how much food to eat.

Monitoring and Modifications: Keep a close eye on developments and health indicators. Over time, sustain weight loss and health gains by making necessary adjustments to the food and exercise regimen.

Support Systems: Seek advice and encouragement from support systems, such as online forums, support groups, or medical experts, in order to sustain long-term success.

Constant Learning: Remain up to date on nutrition guidelines, fitness fads, and new research. Refine and enhance health habits by incorporating new knowledge into daily living.

Flexibility in Lifestyle: Work within the constraints of the Atkins Diet. To maintain sustainability, modify the diet to fit shifting demands, preferences, and health requirements.

Wellness of the Emotions and Mind: Give your emotions and mind first priority. Healthy coping strategies, enough sleep, and stress reduction enhance general wellbeing and help people maintain their weight.

People can keep the weight loss and health advantages of the Atkins Diet by adopting these tactics and applying them to their everyday lives. Long-term weight control and general health success depend heavily on mindfulness, consistency, and a balanced diet and exercise regimen.

Strategies for Lifelong Wellness

Within the framework of the Atkins Diet, holistic approaches to health and well-being are strategies for lifetime wellness:

Long-Term Mindset: Adopt a lifelong dedication to well-being instead of concentrating just on immediate objectives. Consider the Atkins Diet as a long-term lifestyle option as opposed to a band-aid solution.

Nutrient-dense foods, such as lean proteins, healthy fats, and non-starchy vegetables, should be prioritized in order to maintain a balanced diet. For long-term health benefits, make sure your food selections are high-quality and varied.

Frequent Physical Activity: Include in routines that combine strength training, flexibility training, and aerobic activities. Regular exercise bolsters general health and enhances the benefits of food.

Develop mindful eating habits by controlling portion sizes, being aware of your hunger cues, and refraining from emotional eating. It's possible to have a positive relationship with food and remain mindful.

Constant Learning and Adaptation: Keep up with the latest developments in fitness, nutrition, and health. In light of new information, modify and enhance the Atkins Diet strategy to promote long-term wellness.

Prioritize your emotional well-being by controlling your stress, obtaining enough sleep, and fostering wholesome connections. Overall wellness is greatly influenced by emotional well-being.

Regular Health Check-Ups: Make an appointment for routine medical examinations with medical specialists to receive examinations, screenings, and advice on preserving good health.

Support Systems: To get inspiration, motivation, and to share experiences on the path to wellness, connect with your support systems, whether they be friends, family, or medical groups.

Flexibility and Adaptability: Within the parameters of the Atkins Diet, be adaptable and give yourself permission to make changes in response to personal requirements, changing conditions, and changing health objectives.

People following the Atkins Diet can promote lifetime wellness by incorporating these techniques into their regular routines. A comprehensive strategy that incorporates mental health, physical activity, mindfulness, healthy eating, and lifelong learning promotes long-term health advantages and general wellbeing.

Sustainability of Atkins Lifestyle

To guarantee the Atkins lifestyle's long-term viability and success, sustainability requires a number of crucial components, including:

Lifelong Commitment: Accept the Atkins Diet as a long-term lifestyle option as opposed to a band-aid fix. This mental adjustment encourages long-term benefits and consistent adherence.

Realistic and pragmatic: Make sure the Atkins Diet is easy to follow on a daily basis. Customize the strategy to each person's preferences while keeping it reasonable and doable for long-term viability.

Flexibility Within Framework: Give the Atkins framework some leeway. While adhering to its fundamental principles, modify the diet to suit shifting preferences, requirements, and lifestyles.

Holistic Approach: Adopt a holistic approach to health that includes exercise, mental health, and general lifestyle behaviors in addition to dietary modifications.

Make Mindful meal Selections: Make mindful meal selections by emphasizing complete, nutrient-dense foods and keeping an eye on portion sizes and hunger signals. This method encourages a positive connection with eating.

Consistent Exercise Schedule: An essential component of the Atkins lifestyle is continuing to engage in frequent physical activity. This promotes general wellbeing, physical fitness, and weight control.

Ongoing Education: Remain up to date on nutritional facts, health trends, and the most recent research. Apply fresh insights to the Atkins way of life to ensure sustainability and ongoing progress.

Support and Accountability: Seek out sources of encouragement, counsel, and accountability for your wellness journey, such as online communities, friends, and family.

Honoring Progress: Recognize and commemorate accomplishments made possible by the Atkins lifestyle. Acknowledging accomplishments encourages sustained adherence and strengthens healthy behaviors.

People may make sure that the Atkins lifestyle is still feasible, useful, and beneficial in promoting long-term health, wellness, and weight management by including these sustainability methods into their daily routine.